BECOMING THAT GUY

BECOMING THAT GUY

An interventional cardiologist's stories from the cath lab

Brian Herman

ASHWOOD
PUBLISHING

Copyright © Brian Herman 2026

All rights reserved. Apart from as permitted by Australian copyright law, no part of this work may be reproduced by any means without the permission of the author. Contact the publisher for information.

ISBN-paperback: 978-1-7641254-8-2
ISBN-epub: 978-1-7641254-9-9

Published by Ashwood Publishing, Cradoc, Tasmania.
ashwoodpublishing.com.au
info@ashwoodpublishing.com.au

A catalogue record for this work is available from the National Library of Australia.

Cover by Getcovers

The work of Ashwood Publishing is nurtured by the beautiful country of the Melukerdee people in the Huon Valley in southern Lutruwita / Tasmania. We acknowledge and pay respect to the traditional owners and continuing custodians of this place.

To
Daniel and Justin

PREFACE

There are many medical memoirs in the world. Doctors have written memoirs about their times in surgical specialties, in paediatrics, general medicine, obstetrics and gynaecology, trauma surgery, et cetera, et cetera. But when I searched, I could find nothing about my subspecialty, interventional cardiology, which uses a variety of devices to operate on a beating heart with an awake patient, even in the midst of a heart attack. Maybe I missed it, I don't know. Given the importance of this specialty and the prevalence of cardiac disease, I think this is a field worth writing about.

I have two aims in writing this book. One is to tell real-life stories of interventional cardiology, the field I have practised these past four decades. Certain details may have been slightly altered to protect patient confidentiality, but all of these stories are true. The stories illustrate a side of this profession, my life's work, that is exciting, rewarding, and terrifying all at once. Every interventionalist experiences all of these emotions throughout their career. Fear and doubt are pervasive in this profession, standing alongside skill and confidence. Each case ends with an outcome serving to teach lessons for future cases. I am hopeful that the reader will gain a further appreciation of the field. Within the stories, the arc of my life is played out, beginning on one side of the globe, and ending up somewhere that I could not have imagined when it all began. This, too, is part of the tale.

The second reason to write this book is to educate. When I was a child growing up in the United States, there was a clothing store in New York called Syms that ran a regular television commercial espousing the value and quality of their product. But it was the punchline that stayed with me: 'An educated consumer is our best customer.' That's what they were selling. If you were smart enough, discerning enough, you would see the value of their products.

I have used that line on many patients over the years. An educated consumer is our best customer. I like an educated patient. It makes speaking with them, regardless of the problem, easier. I recognize that this is not a black-and-white issue. I cannot and do not expect that an average 'customer' will ever understand all the intricacies of this subspecialty. Nevertheless, if the reader can learn anything from me about this field while reading these stories, I have satisfied a portion of my goals. I want to teach. Within the context of the book, I have included a bit of a primer on the field of cardiology, if for no reason other than to make it 'easier' for me in the story telling, and for the reader to understand. Many of these stories may also be confronting. I hope the reader can accept all of these obstacles in order to learn why this profession is both rewarding and terrifying all at the same time.

People still die from heart attacks. Doctors cannot stop this from happening, regardless of their skills. The sudden nature of massive heart attacks can be catastrophic. Without any warning, a seemingly well individual can face death in less than 60 seconds. Yet so much has changed since Andreas Gruentzig's simple balloon dilatation of a coronary artery on a 40-year-old man in 1977. In my professional career, I have been privileged to have witnessed and participated in the evolution of this specialty. It is a unique career: operating on an awake patient inside a beating heart. Yes, the patient is awake while all of this takes place. And the heart never stops.

It still amazes me today that we are able to access the heart through a tiny incision, pass wires and other devices inside the heart, operate while it is beating … and that it works.

CONTENTS

Preface vii

Prologue 1

Chapter 1 Just a procedure 5

Chapter 2 First case 13

Chapter 3 The heart: a primer 25

Chapter 4 Experience 36

Chapter 5 The day-to-day 49

Chapter 6 The cath lab 61

Chapter 7 So long ago 74

Chapter 8 How did I get into this? 89

Chapter 9 The break 107

Chapter 10 The start of something new 120

Chapter 11 Finding a new home 130

Chapter 12 Teacher 139

Chapter 13 Reputation 154

Chapter 14 On call 164

Chapter 15 Galle 173

Chapter 16 Complications 185

Chapter 17 Home stretch 201

    Acknowledgements 213

    Glossary 215

PROLOGUE

I had just graduated from medical school, moving to a new city to begin what was to be an arduous and challenging career journey. My first rotation as an intern was in the cardiology unit. I cannot emphasize strongly enough how little new graduates knew about clinical medicine. Each year, following graduation ceremonies from medical schools around the country, those more senior would joke that it was the worst time to be admitted into the hospital as a patient. Having a new graduate as your junior doctor was not ideal! This is true, despite what TV medical dramas may depict as to the skill and knowledge of students and interns. Maybe things have changed over the past four decades (although I have my doubts), but I was an all-honours graduate, and I did not know a thing about taking care of patients, despite having followed doctors around for two years on the hospital ward. The first time I was asked to evaluate a patient having chest pain on the cardiology unit, I told the nurse to give the patient some paracetamol, a nonspecific pain treatment. I was too frightened to give a 'real' drug. I was okay with writing orders for Mylanta. That was about it. Rounds were done daily, orders were written, tests were scheduled. No days off for my first month on service. Just learning the routine.

One day, during that first month working on the cardiology ward, I was sitting at the nurses' station writing patient notes, when an urgent yell came down the hall, emanating from a nurse outside a patient's room. No beeper. Just a yell to start running. I quickly entered the room to find an unresponsive female patient. I felt for a pulse and took out my stethoscope to listen for … whatever one listens for. I heard nothing. I felt nothing. She was out. Totally unresponsive.

While I was considering what I should be doing next, the senior resident came bounding into the room pushing the crash cart. He immediately opened the patient's gown and turned on the defibrillator. The gel was rubbed onto her chest, the paddles placed, and the shock delivered. Her heart started beating again. It was the first time I had ever seen that happen. While these devices are commonly used now in the community, even by those unfamiliar with the electrical system of the heart, decades ago you did need to know a thing or two before turning on such a machine. She gradually regained consciousness as he was simultaneously barking a series of orders to the nurses.

I was standing in the room in the same spot as when I entered. The nurses were quickly moving about doing the things he had asked, preparing the patient to be moved to the coronary care unit. I had no clue what to do. I did not know what just happened. I did not, could not comprehend how he knew to do what he had just done. How did he do that? How did he know? The gap in our respective 'knowledge' seemed a very, very wide one.

For much of my life I had wandered aimlessly, wondering what direction I should take. Other than having my degree, with years of training in front of me, I truly had no idea where this was taking me. That day would change everything. For on that day, one thing

Prologue

became crystal clear. That guy who came crashing into that room, taking charge and saving that life – I was going to be that guy. When no one else would know what to do, I was going to know.

Over forty years later, I look back on that moment with grateful satisfaction and hope that maybe, just maybe, I became that guy. These are some of my stories.

CHAPTER 1
Just a procedure

The art of simplicity is a puzzle of complexity.

— Douglas Horton

The year is 1990. The time is 1 a.m. Not for the first time, nor far from the last, I am wearily standing in the emergency department, this time with a 47-year-old man suffering from crushing chest pain. He is sweaty, cold to touch, and unable to breathe. His blood pressure is extremely low, 80/50, and his blood oxygen levels have fallen far below that which is compatible with life. His electrocardiogram (ECG) is diagnostic for a sudden occlusion or blockage of one of the three major arteries supplying heart muscle. The unfolding damage to the heart is already extensive. This clinical condition is known as cardiogenic shock. He is trying to die. Even now, in 2025, his prognosis for survival would be, at best, fifty-fifty. More than thirty years ago, the likelihood of survival would have been less than 15 per cent. In these intervening years, much has progressed in the world of cardiology, the clinical specialty which deals with matters of the heart. At least in the physical sense.

For most patients around that time, medication alone was administered to try to reduce the risk of death from the sort of extensive event that was unfolding in this gentleman. This time, the drugs had failed. What was there to do? Angioplasty (explained below) during an acute heart attack was only then being discussed as an option. Given the uncertainties present, performing angioplasty on a patient who was dying in cardiogenic shock was even more of a risk. A man just 47 years old. Given his poor prognosis without successful treatment, I decided to take him to our operating theatre, known as the cardiac catheterization lab or 'cath lab', in order to open this completely blocked, or occluded, vessel, in the hopes of preserving his dying heart muscle, and thus, extending his life. Despite its complexities, after hours had passed, I had been successful in opening the offending artery, although the damage to his heart was already extensive. He left the cath lab with a mechanical ventilator to assist his breathing, along with numerous intravenous drugs.

I had also inserted a device called an intra-aortic balloon pump, to further assist function of a failing heart. This is a very large balloon placed in the aorta, the largest artery of the body. The balloon extends from the top of the chest through the length of the abdomen. When the heart contracts, the balloon quickly deflates so as not to impede blood flow throughout the body. When the heart is at rest the balloon quickly inflates, acting as a second 'pump' to move blood into the arms, legs – well, everywhere – and into the coronary arteries and cerebral vessels (those going to the brain). It is used when patients are in serious trouble, both to support coronary flow and to aid in patients, like this gentleman, who are in cardiogenic shock: when blood pressure is extremely low and cardiac function becomes incompatible with life.

The gentleman was moved to the intensive care cardiac unit, and I made it home in the wee hours of the morning. I was woken by phone calls over the next two hours keeping me abreast of his condition. He remained hospitalized for a couple of weeks, and almost miraculously, he lived and walked out of the building. His heart was quite damaged, and within the next two years, he was to undergo a cardiac transplant. I continued to follow him for the next few years. He had done remarkably well. I considered this to be a successful outcome in a patient near death. Thousands more cases were to follow. Most with good outcomes, but many not.

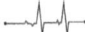

Prior to 1990, the treatment for acute cardiac events had already undergone a major transition. In the 1960s, management of such patients was basically confined to pain control and bed rest. Following decades of research, by the mid-1980s, medication (thrombolytics) was made available to dissolve blood clots in arteries, revolutionizing the treatment for major heart attacks. However, something else was happening that would change the course of cardiovascular medicine.

In 1977, Andreas Gruentzig, a German-born cardiologist, had performed the first balloon dilatation of a coronary artery while working in Berne, Switzerland. Without the use of a general anaesthetic, reaching the heart by advancing coronary catheters via the femoral artery, Gruentzig proved that obstructed blood vessels could be opened by applying physical pressure to the 'blockage' inside the lumen (the inner diameter where the blood itself flows) of the vessel. This, the seminal moment in what came to be known as coronary angioplasty, had taken several years of innovation and invention to reach. Before approaching the coronary vessels, Gruentzig, initially trained as a radiologist, started with dilatation of larger, more peripheral blood vessels in the leg. But with the opening of a coronary artery using an inflatable balloon catheter, the world of cardiovascular disease treatment would be altered forever. A new 'procedure', seemingly so simple yet so elegant and complex, was born.

Traditional cardiac surgery requires the use of general anaesthetics, opening of the chest by cutting through and spreading the sternum, and stopping the heart's beating motion to achieve the goal of 'fixing' the problem. This is done by the construction of conduits, new pathways or 'pipes' using either veins or arteries taken from other sites of the body, to move blood around the blockage, that is, bypassing the blockage. Angioplasty, however, involves operating on awake patients, using local anaesthesia only, accessing the heart via the femoral (leg) or radial (wrist) artery with pieces of long hollow plastic tubing referred to as catheters. All the equipment, such as balloons and stents, are moved through the catheters to hopefully achieve the outcome we all desire.

Early failures were quite common. While his first angioplasty was completely successful, his second was not, and the patient would ultimately require open heart surgery. But it was Gruentzig's belief that it was possible to avoid surgically opening the chest of a patient by 'fixing' arteries with a device that would expand the coronary blood vessel to its original size, physically altering the architectural structure of the artery. Not only would this avoid the long recovery phase of open chest surgery, but the procedure could be done without general anaesthesia, avoiding the known complications of that alone.

Coronary angioplasty was to spawn a whole new subspecialty

in cardiology, referred to specifically as *interventional cardiology*. This is distinguished from general cardiology, in which the technical skills of coronary angioplasty are not needed or utilized. Those of us who trained to do invasive procedures, along with mechanical interventions on blood vessels and valves (plus a number of other structural problems not included here) came to be called interventional cardiologists, or interventionalists. Since the inception of angioplasty, literally millions of patients have undergone this procedure. The rewards to the patient can be immeasurable, but the risks involved can be of equal magnitude. A large part of the role of the interventionalist is weighing those risks against the rewards. In the past thirty years, thousands upon thousands of research papers have been published, having enrolled hundreds of thousands of patients in varying trials, attempting to tease out these risks and benefits. Who obtains the greatest benefit? When do the risks outweigh such a benefit? I think it fair to say that this has not been a simple undertaking.

The heart is essentially a motor. When working normally, it is firing on all eight cylinders. When damaged, the number of 'cylinders' functioning becomes diminished, leading to a constellation of clinical problems. There is an old joke about the garage mechanic who asks the interventionalist why he makes so much more money than him, since they both essentially work on motors. The interventionalist replies, 'Try working on it while it's running!' This is why I have believed this field to be a unique area of medicine. In these coronary interventions we work on a beating heart, while it is running, with patients who are wide awake and speaking with us during the operation. Yes, you heard that correctly, while the patient is awake.

The progress that has been made in the field in my professional lifetime is staggering. It took years after Gruentzig performed that first angioplasty for its use and acceptance around the world to evolve. The equipment needed to be manufactured and delivered. One had to acquire such equipment from one of the few companies producing the gear. Unlike the interconnected world we live in today, where information is disseminated worldwide within minutes to days, early teaching seminars required travelling long distances to even see such a procedure done. The risks were relatively large in the earliest years, with even Gruentzig having a failure rate over 30 per cent. Such failures would frequently turn into emergency open heart operations, which by being an emergency, increased the mortality risks to the patient. In a busy cardiac hospital, it was common to see such emergencies occur on a fortnightly basis. Only the most 'straightforward' cases were done in the era of balloon angioplasty. If the coronary anatomy was complex, it was rare to try the use of a balloon to fix it.

Fast forward to today. Once armed with a few simple drugs, a blood thinner, and an inflatable balloon to open vessels, this subspecialty within cardiology has evolved into an area of care unrecognizable over forty years ago. Its aim is to fix a range of structural problems in a minimally invasive way.

For decades the dominant entry site was at the crease of the upper thigh, where the femoral artery can be felt. While this access site is still used today, with the advent of smaller devices the majority of cases can be done through the radial artery located in the wrist, allowing patients to get out of bed and walk much earlier, while keeping bleeding to a bare minimum. The initial access through the skin is done with the help of a local anaesthetic. The catheter that reaches the coronary circulation is used both to inject the dye used to 'see' the artery, and to deliver the equipment, if and when it is necessary.

The size of the equipment introduced into the body is 30–50 per cent smaller in diameter than it was thirty years ago, also mitigating bleeding risks. We have moved from balloons to stents (a metallic scaffold of sorts), with more than five generations of stent technologies and dozens of iterations of stent design behind us. Initially a wire is passed into the artery, crossing the blockage, followed by delivery of balloons or stents. The wire functions as the rail to move the balloons and stents on. These wires are quite thin, the equivalent of perhaps 3–5 human hairs in diameter (a third of a millimetre), each with different properties. Stents, left within the artery, are effectively a metallic alloy created to scaffold the vessel once opened, to maintain patency (flow). They are tiny: no thicker than 80 microns (one micron equals one thousandth of a millimetre). The stents are crimped on a deflated balloon. When stents were first released, they were crimped on the balloon by hand. That was the job of the primary operator. It didn't take long before manufacturers performed this task in the factory, making it less likely that the stent would simply fall off the balloon! Once in the appropriate location, the balloon can be inflated, opening up the stent. The balloon is then deflated and removed, leaving the expanded or deployed stent in place.

These slicker, smaller balloons and stents allow device therapy to reach anatomy once thought too difficult to reach. Blood vessels are not straight. They have lots of curves and turns. Early devices could not negotiate many of these anatomic variations, yet now, with advanced designs, almost anywhere is 'reachable' for a skilled operator. Even arteries that have been totally blocked for years can frequently now be opened, thanks to technologic and materials advancement. Drug therapies used both during and after the procedure have been game changers as to long term success.

The technique in itself is fascinating, all done under x-ray guidance with mild sedation given at the discretion of the operator (as well as the wishes of the patient). During these procedures, as we watch the operation unfold, it can take the feel of a video game, watching the x-ray screen while manually manipulating the tools. Many a time, I have looked down at the patient lying there, staring at the chest, only to remind myself I am actually in there, inside there, moving all of this stuff around! To an experienced operator, those large arteries we enter are quite strong, or robust. That is to an experienced operator. Someone with little knowledge can easily damage even the largest and strongest vessels in the circulatory system. As arteries become smaller in size, the hand movements, the technical skills become finer, gentler. Damaging coronary-size arteries takes little more than a push, or a tap on the shoulder effort, if done in the wrong place. Gaining adequate experience is measured in a thousand rounds of practice.

The brief outline here does not fully do justice to how this specialty has evolved. Presenting a bit of this history through the subsequent stories is to tell the reader what this life has been like. It's an intense life filled with rewards, stress, punishing hours, successes that save lives, failures that end them – from boredom to exhilaration. So many terrific moments. And so many heart-breaking ones. After many decades since my start, I have witnessed it all.

CHAPTER 2
First case

We learn wisdom from failure much more than from success.

— Samuel Smiles

Before I had a bicycle, there was the tricycle. What we called a trike. It had belonged to my older cousins and begun the time-honoured process of being passed along to younger family members. It was my turn. I loved that trike. Two back wheels and a single front, it was mine to use in the playground where I grew up. It was taller than the average tricycle that would be manufactured in the years to come, and for now, before I would pass it along, it was mine. But like all things in childhood, it was eventually time to move up in style and speed. To the 'bike'. Everyone knows that the transition to two wheels takes a little practice, but once mastered will last a lifetime. And again, most also know that the transition to the bike is frequently done with the help of a parent. With me, it was my dad. Running alongside the bike, holding onto the seat, gradually releasing. So much comfort in knowing that your dad is right there to guide you until you get it. And then he is needed no more. You are growing up.

In cardiology training, too, I had always been under the watchful, guiding eye of someone more senior. You might say they were holding that seat. Following graduation from medical school, I had spent the better part of the past six years preparing myself for this moment. Years of working weekends and nights during residency and fellowship. Responsibilities increasing with the progression of seniority and knowledge. Years of having a second job to afford to raise a family, working those weekends in emergency rooms or intensive care units (ICUs) when not on call. All behind me now. It was time to begin. It was time that I would ride on my own, no one holding the seat.

It is both a wondrous and a stressful transition, moving from trainee to consultant. Having watched, participated, studied, learned, practiced, always knowing you are supported. Always aware that a senior cardiologist is there to help. Always protected to a degree from making errors, mistakes, mishaps. Someone there to bail you out when things are not going as smoothly as you had hoped for. But those days were now in the past. The training was done, and I was now a consultant. The realization struck me that from now on all the successes as well as all the failures were mine to own. No longer supervised. No one to call for help when things went awry. It is what one works towards. To be an independent interventionalist who is respected by peers and patients alike.

When the moment arrived for me, I can only describe my feelings as a conflicted mix of calm and nervous fear. It is not as if I didn't know what I was doing. I was confident as an operator, and comfortable in the surroundings of a cardiac 'cath' lab, the theatre in which intracardiac procedures are done. Proud to take up my first position as a consultant. Yet somehow, standing in the lab, about to do my first case independently, a certain anxiety also swept over me. I had moved my family to an entirely new city to take up this job. I was an unknown entity to all those who I now found myself surrounded by in the hospital. I had new partners in the practice and colleagues who were completely unknown to me. New position, new city, new colleagues, new partners. Much to prove, we tell ourselves. I was calmed, however, by knowing that at least this first case, my first independent 'procedure', was to be 'straightforward' – a term I would forever afterwards associate with 'watch out'.

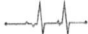

The patient, Mr Roberts, was a gentleman in his fifties who had been complaining of worsening angina, a symptom usually described as chest discomfort with effort, commonly caused by a progressive narrowing of the coronary arteries, the so called 'fuel lines' of the heart. It is rather amusing to me now, looking back, that I thought this was an 'elderly' man – the limited, and yet persistent, perspective of the young.

To briefly explain the basics, as our blood vessels become more obstructed or clogged with plaque material, blood flow to the heart muscle is progressively compromised, causing a constellation of symptoms, the most common of these being referred to as angina. When symptoms come on more frequently with less effort, we use the phrase *unstable angina*. Mr Roberts had presented with a typical and classic case of unstable angina. The diagnostic procedure chosen was to proceed to the cath lab, where an invasive investigation was performed to discover the anatomic cause of his symptoms.

The investigation involved manipulating a catheter inside the blood vessels of Mr Roberts's body to ultimately reach his heart, whereby an iodinated contrast dye was injected directly into the coronary blood vessels to visualize the arteries. These vessels or arteries cannot normally be seen under x-ray without using a contrast agent. A large coronary artery is 4–7 mm, with the average size being no more than 3 mm. (Compare that to the aorta, which is around ten times the size at 25–35 mm. A dilated aorta can grow well beyond 50 mm.) Needless to say, the coronary blood vessels are relatively small given the demands placed upon them. The coronary vessels that we see are those that we can mechanically fix. But as described in chapter 3, these vessels branch off as one moves downstream, much as a tree branches as it grows further from its roots. Ultimately these arteries become a size not visible to the naked eye. We refer to these vessels as the *microvasculature*. And there are tens of thousands of them. These vessels are currently unable to be 'fixed' mechanically and are targeted by medication alone. It is the so-called *macrovasculature* – those arteries that we can see – that is the target of our interventions, whether it be by open heart surgery (referred to also as bypass surgery) or angioplasty.

So, the plan for my first solo procedure on Mr Roberts, *my* patient, was to proceed with a coronary angiogram, outline the anatomic problem, and make a decision as to the next course of action in the hope of 'fixing' this potentially serious and life-threatening clinical problem. This was all considered routine, if not without risk. As we were prepping and draping him to maintain sterility, I was quietly confident, if not a bit nervous, joking with the staff, patient and radiographers, all of whom were new to me. I had done all of this hundreds of times in training. Next, I asked the patient how he was doing.

'Fine, doc. Hope you had a good sleep last night!' Not the first nervous response I would get from someone in his position.

'No worries, Mr Roberts. I always have a couple shots of whiskey before I start to keep my hands from shaking,' I said, as I showed him my feigned tremor. This was a sight gag I would use for years to come to get the patient comfortable and relaxed as I would always see the smile come to their face. I could not help thinking of my recently deceased father, who always went for the laugh. 'Just getting ready to get started, Mr Roberts …'

Things went quickly from there and Mr Roberts was discovered to have a 99 per cent blockage in one of the three major arteries in his heart. Definitely, this would need to be fixed. His other vessels were perfectly normal, as was his heart function. This was *the* perfect first case: one blockage in an otherwise excellent heart. The blockage itself was discrete, covering a length no more than 10 mm. This was the perfect case for an angioplasty.

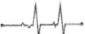

Now I must pause the story for a moment and place this case in a historical context. In today's world, we would absolutely move towards the deployment of a coronary stent. As previously noted, this is a metal scaffold placed in the artery to maintain patency, or openness. Stents have been in common use since the early 1990s, avoiding the many complications associated with balloon angioplasty. In the 1980s, before the routine use of stents, angioplasty was done with a balloon. The balloon would be inflated to 'crack' the cholesterol plaque, then deflated, and finally removed.

Balloon inflation times would vary, but routine inflations were performed for one to two minutes to allow the plaque to become modified and reshaped. Following the removal of the balloon, the vessel would ideally remain the size that it was inflated to, while suffering some modest trauma to the vessel itself. With time, the vessel trauma would heal and leave a nice open artery. At least in theory. It was a theory that worked often, but complications were common. Vessels could tear, rupture, or simply recoil back to their original blocked size. Quickly. It is often forgotten that while that first coronary balloon angioplasty was performed without any problems, a month later Gruentzig would fail on his second patient, who would subsequently require open heart surgery. I often wonder, if patient one had been a failure, would further attempts been as feasible? Fortunately, for the world at large, these techniques would continue to evolve from that day. Remember, too, that this 'procedure' is done on awake patients. Mild sedation may be offered, but it has been an important part of angioplasty to have the patient conscious enough to tell the operator how they are feeling. The feedback is an important part of providing the operator with additional information as the cases progress.

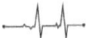

After I told Mr Roberts of our findings, I assured him that for single artery disease, balloon angioplasty was the procedure of choice in most cases, as opposed to having open heart bypass surgery. His was a classic presentation of increasing angina with the perfect anatomic substrate for balloon angioplasty. The perfect first case.

The necessary equipment was brought to the table. I began. I changed the catheter to another type that is specifically designed for angioplasty, and, advancing the angioplasty balloon, the site of blockage was easily crossed. I inserted and inflated the balloon with ease. All according to plan. No sooner had the balloon been inflated than Mr Roberts picked up his head and said to me, 'It's not going very well, is it, doc?' I still remember those precise words many decades later. Naturally, with the balloon inflated, he may have been having some chest discomfort, since the balloon blocks flow temporarily.

'No,' I responded, 'everything is going perfectly smoothly,' as my eyes scanned all the images, blood pressure and ECG tracings on our monitors. Now, what I don't remember decades later is this next time gap. But I am pretty certain that within two seconds of my 'no', his head flopped back onto the table while his eyes rolled into his head ... and he arrested. A glance at the ECG showed him to be in ventricular fibrillation, essentially stopping his heart from beating. I immediately deflated the balloon and called simultaneously for the paddles to be placed to deliver the electrical shock to his chest to restart his heart. (Again, such devices are now seen in supermarkets, airports, and sporting arenas, but were confined to cardiac units then.)

One, two, three ... five shocks delivered, and his heart finally recovers spontaneous electrical activity. While all of this is transpiring, he is placed on a ventilator to mechanically breathe for him. A code blue has been called, sending in the cavalry from the hospital to assist in resuscitation of the patient, which in a cath lab is generally confined to managing the airway. The response to a code blue is usually associated with the arrival of at least a dozen people, a mix of anaesthetists, junior physicians and nurses. As the room is filling up with people, Mr Roberts' heart rhythm had returned, but his blood pressure was reading 50/30 – not compatible with life. A quick injection of dye in the artery I am working on reveals it to be completely occluded, with no flow. A myriad of drugs are being administered. Another anatomic site is being prepped so that I can insert an intra-aortic balloon pump to assist his dying heart. I look around this crowded room with all varieties of health professionals assisting in all kinds of activity. I have now given dozens of orders for a variety of reasons to keep this man alive. I am trying to do multiple physical interventions simultaneously. I make repeated attempts to re-establish flow in this occluded artery to no avail. I have a blood thinner and a balloon. That is my toolbox. These are the only tools available to try to reopen and re-establish flow in this artery. (How that toolbox will grow in the ensuing decades!) Despite numerous attempts to reopen this vessel, the artery remains occluded. Mr Roberts is in big trouble. There are now five IV drugs running, a large intra-aortic balloon assist device hanging out of his left leg, and a blood pressure (BP) barely compatible with life. He was just speaking with me … and now he is dying. This is a theme repeated over and over again in many of my stories. The speed at which the tide turns, and the speed at which the response must be made. What was an ideal case for an angioplasty was a catastrophe in the making.

What happened next in this catastrophic complication has stayed with me after these many years. I do not exaggerate. In the midst of the bedlam that I was responsible for creating, I had what I can only call the only out of body experience of my life.

Now, I am not a particularly strong believer in the spiritual world. My thoughts on the matter are ever changing and evolving, very much related to my own aging process. There are many things that occur in nature that we don't have explanations for, but I personally do not feel the need to subsequently leap to some alternative reality theory or some greater spiritual being to explain the inexplicable. I have become far too grounded in scientific principles to reach for the supernatural or mystical. And yet this moment, this event, happened to me. And the sensation, the memory, the moment has stayed with me, even after the thousands of cases to come in my future. With all hell breaking loose in front of me, the thing I could not help but notice was that at this point I was now the only doctor in the room. A room full of supportive personnel looking to me. I was 'that guy' – the only guy in that room who was supposed to know what to do next.

This is what I recall. Everything became very quiet. I heard nothing. Silence. Time seemed to stand still. It was then as if a ghost figure left my body. It looked exactly as I did. When it looked down from where it had floated above, I could literally see myself standing at the table, furiously working to stabilize the patient. It was then that my ghost figure turned to the nurse and said, 'Go get the consultant.' She did not respond. (I'm pretty sure I was the only one aware of the ghost!) This apparition was only present for less than 10 seconds, before it returned and joined my physical self to say, 'You are the consultant!' Calling for a more senior person was what one did during training, fellowship. This was no longer the case. There was no one else to come to the rescue. It was a sobering realization. Yet I knew that I had been trained well, and I knew that I knew what to do.

After over two hours of effort, I managed to stabilize the situation and keep Mr Roberts alive. It was clear that he needed to go for emergency open heart surgery. The angioplasty had failed, and it was the only option.

It is a sickening feeling to admit that you have failed in your attempt to avoid what is now both necessary and dangerous.

With the help of staff, I pushed that trolley, along with multiple IV poles and two large machines attached to the patient, to the elevator and down to the operating theatre, not knowing whether he would survive. And if he did, would he be normal again? Were our resuscitation efforts adequate, enough to avoid other organs of the body being injured, particularly the brain? As I left him in the operating theatre, I was shaken inside. This was my first case, *my first* … It was supposed to be easy.

I spent a very restless evening at home. These early complications weighed heavily on my life, my career. It all happened so quickly. What kind of way was this to 'make a living'? It had taken no longer than a few moments for it to leave its scars. Looking back years later, maybe I was learning an important lesson. That there is never room for complacency in this line of work. The case is not done until it is. On numerous occasions, I have heard the nurse say to the patient that we are almost done. It is to give the patient a sense of ease that, well, all has gone smoothly and we are close to the end. At those moments, I stop, make eye contact with the nurse with my serious 'game face', and give the look of disapproval. Never, never say it is done until it is *done*. It is so common to believe you are finished only to have something happen. It is the suddenness of it all. These are important lessons, but why did I have to learn them during my first case?

The following day, I knew that Mr Roberts had survived the surgery. He would leave the hospital ten days later and would continue his follow-up with one of my colleagues. I felt guilt for many years about what happened. I had seen many patients pass away over my years of training in both general medicine and cardiology. I had spent years 'moonlighting' in emergency rooms where it was common for people to have passed away before they had arrived in the emergency department. I had dealt with families under the worst of circumstances. Families placed in the quiet rooms most often reserved for the delivery of upsetting and life-altering news, that was as sudden as it was unexpected. It was never pleasant. But this was not the same thing; it was very, very different. To be the causative agent in death, or in any major complication, is a different level of responsibility. It weighs on your thoughts, on your life, until you learn to live with this part of the work. Living a life where illness and loss of life is common does something to you. When you're young, life seems endless and full of opportunities and dreams for the future. This world I had entered changes things. You experience up close and personal the end of the dreams that others have lived. There is a 'weight' to it all. With time you become hardened a bit. Not unfeeling, but as if a wall is slowly built between yourself and the emotional pain of those under your care. If you're not careful, this wall begins to creep into your own personal life and create barriers to your own emotional growth. It's not easy to explain to someone who has not experienced this. It is, however, a survival mechanism for those of us who deal with the most acute of diseases. My 'wall' was not even close to being constructed in those early years. The guilt stayed with me.

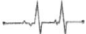

I met Mr Roberts again over ten years later. It was a meeting unplanned and equally unexpected by me. He asked me if I remembered him – for him, an honest question but for me, a question bordering on absurdity. I had never sought him out. If anything, I would have crossed the street to avoid him if the opportunity had arisen. I had lived with this shame and guilt for years, always assuming that he would never want anything to do with me. The shame of 'failure', a bad outcome. The guilt of having nearly ended his life with the simple manipulation of a tiny balloon no larger than 2½ mm. The conviction that he held me responsible for nearly causing his death, for in my eyes, that was the truth.

What he then said to me upon our meeting has stayed with me equally as long as the memory of that first procedure. He thanked me. He thanked me for saving his life, knowing that if this artery had blocked off at home he would have certainly died. The nurses had spoken to him of the lengths I had gone to keep him going, and the professionalism I had shown to all of those working on him. I am thankful for those who upheld me in one of those moments when I most needed support. Perhaps, he believed, without my attendance he would never have survived the day.

I didn't know what to say. All of my shame, my guilt …

I remember feeling flabbergasted at the generosity of his thoughts. At the generosity of the staff who sought not to blame me, but to uphold all that I sought to do. I don't know that the guilt ever went away, but his kindness humbled me more than I can express. It was important. My first case …What a way to start a career.

CHAPTER 3
The heart: a primer

A hospital bed is a parked taxi with the meter running

— Groucho Marx

Before moving on, I thought it appropriate to stop here and do a bit of education. The case histories that I write about can be daunting enough, but by attempting to teach some of the basic material and the language which is frequently used throughout these stories, I hope to provide the reader with the basis to understand what is actually happening during these episodes. And to offer better insight and understanding of both the anatomic features of the heart itself, and the methods used to manage those problems frequently encountered. This is, as best as I can put it, the 'educated consumer is my best customer' chapter.

In general, cardiology is a specialty field of general medicine which concentrates and attends to illnesses that affect the heart. While over the years it has expanded to encompass diseases involving the overall vascular (blood vessel) system, that is, cardiovascular disease, its core remains anchored in those diseases affecting cardiac structure and function. In the Western world of developed economies, cardiovascular disease is far and away the number one cause of death. And in those countries where an affluent middle class began to emerge from widespread poverty in the later 20th century, disease of the heart has grown even faster, to almost epidemic proportions. Its economic impact can be measured in terms of both the costs of modern diagnostic and therapeutic modalities, and the costs of lost work. The emotional costs are more difficult to quantify, yet are there, nevertheless.

Unlike many illnesses which may lead to death or disability in a chronic, slow, and sometimes insidious fashion, heart disease has the capacity to strike with alarming speed. For those who succumb (that is, die) suddenly, the medical term is simple: sudden cardiac death. While statistics are at times difficult to interpret, published data spanning decades have concluded that as many as one-third to one-half of patients who die from cardiovascular disease die suddenly. It is a sobering thought that so many families will discover that this pathology existed in their loved one when the time to respond is too late. What these numbers don't show, however, are those patients who in fact had the warning signs, but did not recognize them, or chose to ignore them. Often the ignoring of symptoms is simply based on fear. The fear and ultimate denial of a problem that one wishes not to face, *despite* having a problem that could well be amenable to being fixed. Sudden, acute, devastating. The emotional toll on those left behind with no preparation for the grieving, nor a chance to reconcile what is to come, is shattering.

It is not always this way, though. Heart disease can behave in a slower and more subtle fashion. Years of symptoms may ensue, with a gradual deterioration of overall functional capacity. In some cardiac patients, the terminal stages can even appear not dissimilar to other end-stage diseases like cancer. Symptoms take the form of weight loss, loss of appetite, muscle wasting, and generalized weakness, making everyday activities increasingly difficult. Over twenty-five years ago, this chronic, slowly progressive loss of function was far more common, a not-infrequent presentation with those suffering from chronic congestive heart failure. In our current era, with the advent of more effective medication and structural interventions, this type of slow, insidious cardiac mortality is less often seen. I, like many others, have never been certain which is preferable, fast or slow. A sudden mortality seems easier on the patient, but harder on the family. Slow deterioration gives families time to adjust, but not very happy times for the patient. One can pontificate on this sobering subject for lengthy periods of time, but if any of it is manageable, fixable, or lightens the load, then that's the job I have chosen.

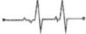

So, what is 'heart disease'? Let's start at the beginning. The heart is amazing, to be certain. A motor, a pump, that never rests and never stops. If you live to be 70 years of age, with an average resting heart rate of 72 beats per minute, it will have contracted more than 3 billion times (noting that the pulse rate is far more commonly elevated than the resting rate). Asleep and awake it goes about its sole job, delivering a blood supply, and nutrients, to all other parts of the functioning body. When demand for flow is increased, such as with an exercising muscle, it's the job of the heart to increase its output to meet the demand. If the demand for blood flow is not met, the muscle would simply fatigue, and physical exertion would end. The heart delivers blood to the kidneys to filter our toxins, to our brain to keep normal neurological processes intact, to our skin to regulate body heat, to our gut to allow it to do the job of food digestion. In fact, without us knowing it, demand from our gut will increase the output of the heart by 25 per cent just by eating a meal. If the heart doesn't respond accordingly, digestion and absorption of food substances won't occur normally. In essence, the sole purpose of the heart is to service the needs of the rest of your body. It is a muscle. A pump. That is all. Yet it is astonishing, nonetheless.

In many respects, it's such a simple organ. It is asked to do one thing and one thing only. It must squeeze. Compare that to the complexities of the central nervous system, or the multiple tasks of the liver or pancreas. With each squeeze (contraction) of the heart, blood is ejected through its various chambers, eventually entering the general circulation. That's it. Its job is done. I have often wondered why so many consider the heart to be the most important organ of the body, given the simplicity of its job. Ancient Greeks, Hebrews, Taoists, Chinese philosophers, all attribute the centre of thoughts and emotions to the heart. The Old Testament references the heart as the centre of wisdom. The New Testament suggests the heart is where thought begins. And of course, ancient texts preceding the time of the Greek empire believed that in this central organ, where visceral pain may be felt, sits the seat of desire. Regardless of your philosophy or belief system, without this perpetually functioning pump, the inevitability of the end of life is near certain.

1. The Engine
There are four cardiac chambers, each possessing different properties, and slightly different types of muscle tissue. When the

heart contracts, it must generate enough pressure to propel blood through the circulation for it to reach the organs of the body. While people typically think solely of the heart's contractile (squeezing) function, the heart *must* also relax. Relaxation doesn't sound like much, but this part of the cardiac cycle is perhaps as important as the contractile one. Without normal relaxation, the chambers cannot fill again. Imagine a muscle, any muscle, that contracts but does not relax. If it were your biceps, perhaps with a powerful contraction, you could curl 50 kg. But without relaxation of the muscle, the arm could not straighten out afterward. Despite its obvious strength, how useless an arm this would be. The relaxation phase of the cardiac cycle, like any muscle, is crucial to its overall function. Like the frozen biceps noted, a contraction not followed by relaxation would not allow it to fill with blood to squeeze again.

The four cardiac chambers are divided into the two halves of the heart. The right heart chambers are called the right atrium and right ventricle; the left heart chambers are called the left atrium and left ventricle. They share a common 'wall' between them, the septum. These two halves are profoundly different from one another despite being attached. The right heart chambers deliver blood to the lungs, and the left chambers to all other areas of the body. The overwhelming burden of pathology, or effectively most of the disease that we concern ourselves with, is seen involving the left heart chambers, with the left ventricle being the site where most of the heavy lifting for moving blood through the circulation is found. This is the most muscular chamber, and the one most commonly affected when patients have heart attacks. Not to minimize the role of the other chambers of the heart, but the preservation of the left ventricle is often the focus of much of our efforts.

This is how the circulation works. Blood will first enter the heart via the right atrium and flow to the right ventricle. It will exit to the lungs, where oxygen is picked up, then return to the left atrium, left ventricle, and then be ejected from the left ventricle into the aorta. From the aorta, this oxygenated blood will disperse throughout the body, via an intrinsic pipeline architecture, to all vital organs and muscle. Once oxygen is extracted from the blood to 'feed' the organs, it will enter into the venous architecture, ultimately returning to the heart to once again enter the right atrium. It is one complex and sophisticated amusement park ride.

2. The Valves
Deployed in between the various chambers of the heart and the general circulation are fibrous structures referred to as heart valves. Think of these as little doors that open and close during the cardiac cycle, allowing blood to flow forward from chamber to chamber, and ultimately into the aorta. The most significant function of these valves is to prevent forward moving blood from going backwards, potentially returning to a chamber it has already exited. Think of going through customs when arriving at the airport. Once you leave the customs area with your baggage, those sliding doors are not letting you go back in. Similarly, once blood exits a chamber in forward flow, there is no going back in. Blood flow moving in the backwards direction, referred to as regurgitant flow, can create major problems. A normal functioning valve allows blood to move forward as it opens and prevents backward flow when it closes, all in timing with the contraction and relaxation phases of the cardiac cycle. Not that complex. Only that, as I have mentioned earlier, it must do this billions of times in a lifetime.

3. The Electrical System

So, we now know that muscle contraction is the core business of the heart. To pump and relax. With little doors opening and closing inside, the flowing blood is kept moving forward from one cardiac chamber to another and into the circulation. Once again, I describe it as a mechanical engine of sorts. Moving parts, like the pistons of an engine, and valves, to prevent leakage. And like an engine, it also has an electrical system. You can buy a brand-new motor, but without some initiating power source, an electrical spark that starts the engine's moving parts, nothing happens.

One of the more fascinating and intricate parts of the heart is its intrinsic power supply and all the subsequent wiring accompanying it. The heart is capable of creating its own 'spark' of sorts, which begins an electrical current that subsequently spreads throughout all cardiac muscle. It is this current that is the stimulant for muscle contraction. Imaging owning a power source, a battery, that never needed recharging. Each time an initiating 'spark' is needed, without fail an electric current is created. And that this capacity to generate an electrical current is performed billions of times, year after year. Never needing to be turned off. Connected to nothing. Simply a self-generating source of electrical energy. This is what the heart is capable of when you are born. The additional electrical connections of the heart are also rather sophisticated, with specialized bundles of wires that conduct these impulses throughout the chambers, leading the cardiac muscle fibres to contract in a coordinated wave, maximizing the heart's ability to move blood throughout the system. When all works according to plan, you have an engine that has a self-perpetuating power source, capable of moving hundreds of millions of litres of blood in a lifetime, providing for all other organs of the body. Impressive.

4. The Fuel Lines

Now let us say you have a brand new eight-cylinder car, the motor in perfect working order, the valves and gaskets functioning normally, accompanying a brand-new battery with state-of-the-art electronics ready to roll. And then someone comes along and dumps sugar in the gas tank. Big trouble. For the final piece missing in our magnificent design of an engine is the fuel lines, with the fuel required to keep it functioning. For those of us with a heart, the fuel itself is blood. Without a blood supply, the heart, like all other organs, would fail. The fuel lines that deliver that blood supply to heart muscle are called the coronary arteries. It is very, very important to note that the blood moving through the cardiac chambers is *not* the primary source of fuel to this cardiac engine. While some of it is used to keep the heart muscle nourished, the blood in the chambers is ultimately destined for delivery elsewhere.

The 'fuel lines' of the heart are a separate circulation, the coronary arteries. These are blood vessels that are literally found sitting on the surface of the heart with their origins found coming off near the beginning of the aorta, the largest blood vessel of the body. As noted in an earlier section, these coronary vessels can be as large as 4–7 mm, gradually tapering in size as these arteries branch off to cover the area of the heart. An average diameter coronary vessel is 2.5–3 mm. Ultimately, they reach a size unseen by the naked eye (less than 0.3–0.5 mm). These tiny vessels, the so-called microvasculature, make up the vast majority of the circulation to cardiac muscle, as is true throughout all of the vascular systems in the body. When coronary blood vessels become 'diseased', a term generally reflecting the build-up of obstructive plaque within the lumen of the artery, this is termed coronary artery disease. It may be mild, moderate, severe, or life threatening in its severity. It may involve one artery, so called single vessel disease, or all arteries and their branches, referred to as multivessel disease. It is the narrowing of these vessels by obstructing plaque that is responsible for the most common symptoms of heart disease, as well as the majority of heart attacks and sudden cardiac death. Pathology of the microvascular system is beyond our current capability to accurately diagnose and, often, to treat. It is the larger vessels, the ones we can see, that have been the target of most of our efforts these past sixty years. Each coronary vessel, as you would expect, has a name, reflecting the anatomic position in the heart. Not to overwhelm the reader, I have yet to mention them, although they are referred to in the stories. And they are listed in the accompanying glossary of terms, a quick reference for those needing a jogging of the memory while reading on.

Simply put, if you have clogged up the fuel lines (the coronaries), even with a perfectly normal engine (our heart muscle), the flow of fuel to that engine is now compromised. This may result in chest discomfort, epigastric (the so-called pit of your stomach) discomfort, heartburn-like symptoms, arm pain, wrist pain, breathlessness, along with a combination of the above, to create a clinical scenario we typically call angina. All of these symptoms are not necessarily indicative of a heart problem, but to a trained ear listening to the whole clinical picture, a suspicion may begin to take shape of a cardiac problem. The very sudden obstruction or complete blockage of one of these vessels is what leads to a heart attack. And with a heart attack, permanent injury or damage to heart muscle is done. Like all things, heart attacks sit on a spectrum of mild to severe. The symptoms alone do not necessarily correlate with the amount of damage done, nor to the life-threatening nature of the anatomic problem. Two people with the exact clinical story will usually have very, very different anatomic problems.

5. Pericardium- the Container

The pericardium is merely a sac that the heart sits in. It has very little to do with cardiac function on a day-to-day basis, and it is rarely noticed unless it is creating a problem. This double-lined structure, to a degree, keeps the heart tethered within the chest and protects it from direct contact with lung tissue. There is a small amount of fluid within this sac that allows a certain degree of 'lubrication', allowing the heart to move freely. The pericardium can become inflamed from viral infections, causing discomfort known as pericarditis. It can also be the site of tumour invasion and other infectious diseases. If this sac fills up with too much fluid, as can occur with inflammation, we may develop a condition called cardiac tamponade, whereby the heart is being squeezed by the surrounding fluid, much like a boa constrictor would squeeze. After all, the sac itself has a limited size already occupied by the beating heart. If too much fluid accumulates, the heart will not have enough room to fill, and cardiac output will fall. Unless the surrounding fluid is removed, the patient will ultimately die. Thus, while generally not thought to have a large role in cardiac disease, the pericardium can create its own set of clinical problems.

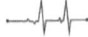

The job of cardiologists is, briefly stated, to attend to any one of a number of these abnormalities of the heart. Following the above format, there are 1) heart muscle, i.e. the engine; 2) coronary arteries, i.e. the fuel lines; 3) the electrical system, i.e. the battery and wiring; 4) the valves themselves, the gaskets that prevent blood from leaking back into a space it has just left; and 5) diseases of the pericardium. There may be a primary problem of the 'engine' itself, where the cardiac muscle is not functioning normally. There may be any number of electrical problems, ranging from electrical irritability causing extra heart beats, to life threatening rhythm disturbances, to a slowly failing 'battery'. Problems can develop with heart valves. They may not open properly. Or when the valve closes, it doesn't create the seal required to prevent backflow, so-called *valvular insufficiency* or regurgitation. And most common of all, the problem of plaque causing obstruction of blood vessels. These occluded fuel lines, which feed the heart, lead to a possible constellation of the symptoms previously noted, and in the extreme, sudden cardiac death.

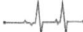

So, in a nutshell, this is the basics of cardiology. The study and treatment of a very sophisticated and sensitive organ whose sole purpose is to move blood through the circulation to serve the needs of all the other organs of the body. Management strategies are varied when pathology of the heart exists. Advances in pharmacology have added so much to patient care, both in treating active disease and in the hopeful prevention of serious pathology. But when patients present with an advanced and unstable clinical scenario, and more is required than medication alone can offer, the role of the interventionalist is frequently called upon.

CHAPTER 4
Experience

Good judgement comes from experience. and experience comes from bad judgement.

— Popular saying

The first time I stepped into, or more appropriately, slid into a white-water kayak, I was in my mid-forties. I had paddled in white-water rafts before, but the kayak was a whole new thing for me. Rolling down white water in a raft versus a kayak is somewhat like the difference between driving a bus and a sports car – a rather different experience to say the least.

I was not a fool, though. I took lots and lots of lessons with experienced guides, paddling rivers that were appropriate for my level. White water ranges from relatively gentle moving water to the roiling rapids seen in YouTube videos, which often appear nearly suicidal. I was not suicidal. I knew my limits. I spent the next couple of seasons in classes while I gradually built up my skills. While I was absolutely not an 'advanced' paddler, I became competent enough to negotiate moderate white water and developed the necessary 'roll' to right myself after the inevitable flipping over that occurs with everyone who steps into one of these boats.

It was the end of the fall season in New England. The leaves had changed colours and the air was crisp as I headed out alone on my final outing of the year. It's a beautiful time of the year to be on the river. Paddling alone is not good practice: anything can happen. But I was determined to go, and I did not have a paddling partner. Great day on the water. River running well, with the classic autumn weather so predictable that time of year. As I approached the final rapids of the day, I was a bit nervous and apprehensive. I had run into trouble with this section of the river before. While I had run it successfully in the past, I thought that this time I would take a slightly different route. And so here I went, careening down the first drop with the waters swirling around me, boulders flying past. I went into the second drop quite quickly and thought I had made it through, when suddenly I hit a flat rock underwater, something I had not seen or appreciated was there in my previous runs through this part of the river. It is vitally important, as you progress in your skills, to know how to 'read' the river. You must see an obstacle coming based on how water is moving. I didn't see it. I hit that rock and immediately flipped. No big deal. I could roll out of it, I told myself. But that didn't allow for the shallowness of the river there and the depth of that particularly large rock. Despite wearing a helmet (fortunately for me), the side of my head hit hard just under the brim of the helmet and above my eye and temple. I was seriously stunned. I vividly remember floating upside down, my body totally relaxed, just listening to the river. Despite the roar of the water when above it, underneath it is quiet. It was quite peaceful. It was a few seconds later that I realized that if I didn't get this boat right-side up, or swim out (in the midst of these rapids), I could drown. I woke up from this place of quietude rather abruptly, realizing the peril I was in. Again, I had enough skill to roll that boat and allow myself to float down the river. My head hurt and I was bleeding. I was glad it was the end of the run with my car only a couple of hundred metres away. There was one guy out on the river at the time, and he paddled up to me to ask if I was okay. He saw me hit. It was obvious to him that I had a bad flip as he watched my body and boat come to an abrupt jarring stop before further cascading down the river. I was fine, I told him, even if my head was sore. I got to my car and loaded the kayak on the roof rack. The drive home was a couple of hours. A rather large bruise would form on my forehead and drape around my eye, but there would be no lasting damage.

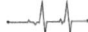

I tell this little vignette of a story as a reminder. Knowledge and skill versus experience: which wins? And when? I had some skills. I had some knowledge. I had even paddled this river multiple times. What I lacked was real life, serious experience. I was alone on that river with few other paddlers about at that time of year. My lack of mastery or expertise while paddling alone was nearly a costly mistake. I was almost knocked unconscious. I didn't read the river. A bad judgement leading to experience. No matter how smart you are, the outcome of doing dangerous things without experience can be the flip of a coin. Or in this case, a kayak.

In chapter 2, I described how I faced my first solo procedure with a mix of confidence and intense fear. The fear was because it is scary as hell to be responsible for someone's life. The confidence came from a belief that I was entering into the profession as one of the 'newest' crop of cardiologists, with state-of-the-art skill and knowledge. Given all the progress in medicine over the previous decades, no other group of physicians had ever come out of training with more information, more preparation. I was, essentially, the latest product of education and mentorship, and thus, by definition, the most informed and perhaps, learned. It is true not just for doctors, but for all professions leaving the world of education and starting a career. Whether you are an accountant, a lawyer, an architect. Any profession that has moved forward based on discovery, innovation, or technological growth finds its newest employees the most educated the world has ever seen. It is a nice thought.

But what we also know is, while a new physician has the latest and the greatest knowledge that modern medicine has to offer, they lack the critical factor of experience. Despite what many would like to believe as to the pure science of medicine, its day-to-day practice is full of events and incidents that are far from black and white. All the science and research and teachings learned cannot prepare anyone to make decisions and choices in so many clinical areas where there is no black-and-white answer. This is the grey zone. And in that zone, where the data are lacking, having been there before can make all the difference in the world. Being there before. This is what we refer to as experience.

I have thought a lot about experience. It is extraordinarily difficult to quantify, or even to truly define. Yes, it does have to do with the time that someone has spent in the field of endeavour, but time itself is only one measuring tool. The variation of interactions, the complexity of the problems encountered, the sheer volume of work delivered, and yes, even the bad outcomes, all contribute to this thing we call experience. I have come to the conclusion that experience is essentially the capacity to 'guess' better. To make decisions based on probability, partly learned and partly lived through. And then ... to guess. Anyone who tells you different is ... mistaken.

And now to the fear. If not yet self-evident, then perhaps after this story it will be. I was to find myself in a position of making important, and sometimes life-threatening decisions based on a vast acquisition of knowledge, yet with modest clinical experience to go alongside it. For the most part, comfort was gained sensing that knowledge alongside skill acquired through training would win out in the end. At least it dampened the fear.

I was confident in my professional skills along with my academic knowledge, as I was with life in general. Reasonably athletic and fit, married with twin sons, my life was sitting on a strong foundation. There were many rocky moments along the way, and would be in the future, but for now I was on solid ground. My training at the University of Pittsburgh in the 1980s had been exemplary. My time there straddled the new frontiers of coronary angioplasty and the older foundations of cardiac haemodynamics, the study of cardiac function and physiology. I have remained indebted to those who trained me. There are very few mentors or teachers that I can recall from my early life, but I do remember my teachers and mentors during my cardiac training, and I remember them well. My training created the solid building blocks of cardiac dynamics that have served me so well over the decades, even as the specialty has grown more complex and increasingly perplexing as the years go on.

Once I left training, the learning curve, if you will, significantly flattened almost immediately. This is again also true for everyone leaving a training program of any kind and entering into the real world. No longer is there someone to teach you daily. The learning comes bit by bit over long periods of time. Sometimes from colleagues, sometimes in conferences. The practical experience of work begins to catch up to the academics you have studied over the years. For some, the academics are entirely lost. Experiences with patients may multiply and mature, but the new learning needed over time may begin to stagnate.

On the other hand, for many true academics, research experience leads to great innovation and breakthroughs, yet their clinical experience dealing with patient-based decisions falters.

My goal was to avoid these two extremes and combine knowledge, skill and clinical experience. Threading that needle, balancing newly acquired knowledge and patient-driven clinical experience, would be the test of a lifetime. Only a few months had passed since my experience with Mr Roberts and his near death on the cath lab table. The guilt that stayed inside me became deeply buried. It is not possible to continue forward in any line of medical practice without pushing such events out of our day-to-day consciousness. I continued to believe, despite what had occurred on that day, that I had been well prepared by being well trained. With a sense of quiet confidence, I would continue on.

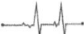

Within the next few months of practice in the hospital, I was asked to see a patient who was in the intensive care unit (ICU) due to low blood pressure. Paul was a man in his mid-sixties who, five days earlier, had had an operation on his oesophagus performed via a thoracotomy incision (through the rib cage). The following post-operative day, he had suffered a heart attack, based on ECG tracings and cardiac enzyme assessment, but had remained clinically stable for days. The cardiac enzyme assessment is a blood test that detects a protein released from damaged heart muscle and serves as a marker for patients who are having a heart attack. I had not met Paul before. He had a history of smoking and significant alcohol consumption through much of his life and was ultimately discovered to have a tumour in his oesophagus. Fortunately for him, it was felt that surgery would be curative, as there was no evidence of spread elsewhere. He had no prior history of cardiac disease, and when I met him in the ICU, he was awake and alert and not complaining of pain or breathlessness.

I was asked to see him predominantly because his blood pressure was running around 90/60, well below his baseline. Any drop of blood pressure to this level is of concern, particularly in a patient who has had both recent surgery and a heart attack. After examining him in the ICU, I elected to do what we refer to as right heart catheterization. Using local anaesthesia only, a catheter is placed through the internal jugular vein in the neck into the right side of the heart and advanced into the pulmonary artery, measuring pressures within each of the cardiac chambers and the pulmonary artery itself. The cardiac output, effectively how much blood the heart is pumping, is then also measured. The purpose of this procedure is to effectively tell the physician if there is a physiological problem with cardiac function. If the problem is truly cardiac, the diagnosis can be made and managed appropriately. If the right heart study is normal, the cause of his low blood pressure is absolutely non-cardiac in origin. It is definitive. I had done literally hundreds of these during my training and was quite comfortable doing this in the ICU, despite the usual setting being in the cath lab.

After explaining the nature of the procedure to Paul, I proceeded with the assistance of the ICU nurse. It all went quite smoothly. As is usual, Paul was wide awake with only a local anaesthetic applied. Once completed, my suspicion of the cause was quickly confirmed. The patient had what is called cardiac tamponade physiology. Fluid had collected within the heart's protective sac, the pericardium, and was squeezing the cardiac chambers, effectively preventing them from refilling effectively after each contraction.

There was now little doubt in my mind that this fluid needed to be 'tapped'(removed). This is done by advancing a needle under the sternum and into the pericardial space, again with the patient awake. Despite having performed this manoeuvre many times over the years, it has always spooked me a bit. You trust the anatomy, yet advancing a needle under the sternum towards the heart itself can be a bit unnerving. Called pericardiocentesis, this is more commonly done in the cardiac cath lab, but having done my fair share of these taps, I set out to do this one in the ICU. As I began to set up for the tap, I carefully explained to the ICU nurse, and to Paul, all that was transpiring. I explained all the initial findings based on the right heart study and what to expect as we moved forward. It has always been in my nature to teach, and at least this was a subject I felt very secure in. And so, I went about teaching the ICU nurse. As for Paul, I didn't think he was in the best of positions to be a student. I suspect he just wanted it done and over with.

All went smoothly. As I slid the needle up and under the sternum, I quickly reached the pericardium without incident. I was then able to aspirate fluid from the pericardial space. His intracardiac pressures normalized and his cardiac output increased. His BP returned to its original baseline. He felt well. The diagnosis was accurate, and the management was curative. With lots of self-satisfaction, as I was establishing myself in my new job, I walked out of the room to write my notes on the patient chart. A good feeling. I had used a specialized skill set in an ICU setting where rarely would such a skill be utilised … Yeah, a good feeling.

That good felling would last for no longer than 60 seconds. As I was writing my notes, the patient crashed. No blood pressure. CPR was commenced. Code blue was called.

As I watch a dozen people answering the code, my mind is racing. What is happening? How could he crash following a successful pericardiocentesis? What have I done? The surgeon who performed his thoracotomy days earlier immediately arrives. Suddenly he takes a surgical blade and opens the left chest in between two ribs, and a litre of blood comes pouring out onto the bed. Unable to see the bleeding site, the surgeon keeps his hand in the opening as the patient is immediately wheeled out of ICU into an operating theatre with his chest open.

There I stand. Alone. One moment feeling modestly heroic; the next the culprit to another potential death. Did I lacerate an artery during the needle puncture? Did I lacerate a coronary vessel? Did I puncture the right ventricle causing literally, a hole in his heart with bleeding directly into his chest cavity? Clearly, I'm a witness and an agent to a catastrophe. The cause is unclear. But my culpability is obvious, at least to me.

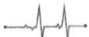

One of the peculiar and uncomfortable parts of this job is that even when bad, horrible, brutal outcomes are occurring in the midst of the working day, you simply continue on. Well, maybe not simply, but continue on you do. The volume of work, the number of patients, the never-ending responsibility of clinical work, mean you must continue to move through the day as if nothing catastrophic has occurred. The next patient wants and deserves your attention. Over the years, I have been involved with scores of procedural complications, and regardless of what happens, you never just put down your pen and your stethoscope and say 'I am done for today.' To do so would create a domino effect on all those others who require time and energy of you. Given what can transpire as a result of interventional complications, it seems insane to just keep going. Just doesn't seem to be a mentally healthy thing to do. Yet that's exactly what you do. Perhaps it is one of the reasons that over the years, all of us in the profession have become 'case-hardened'. Too many days when the luxuries of pausing and reflecting on events are skipped over to serve the many. Perhaps it's merely an emotional survival mechanism. I don't know for certain. I do know, however, that when I speak of my personal life versus my professional clinical one, my voice, my thoughts, my emotional overlay are very, very different.

And so, as I was to learn, my day needed to continue forward, while my thoughts were yet again full of guilt and anxiety, not knowing what had happened or what the ultimate outcome would be. Hours passed waiting to hear from the operating theatre. What had I done to cause this patient to literally bleed out?

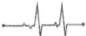

That same afternoon, I was in my office seeing patients when the surgeon finally called. He had opened the chest and, alongside a cardiac surgeon, had inspected the surgical field. They were unable to find any site of bleeding. Despite what had obviously happened in the ICU, there was no indication where the blood had been coming from. After forty-five minutes, they elected to take him off the table, since there was no obvious bleeding site. Chest tubes were placed in both the right and left sides of the thorax and they closed his chest back up.

Thirty minutes after arriving in the recovery room, suddenly both chest tubes filled with blood. There was no stopping this now. Within a minute, Paul was gone. Despite visually looking for a site of bleeding with an open chest, a source was not found. The surgeon was unable to offer an explanation when he called me. With all this effort, it remained unclear as to what had happened.

A week later, the post-mortem report was finished. The cause was apparent. The patient had suffered a full thickness posterior (back wall of the heart) transmural infarction (heart attack) four days prior to the pericardiocentesis, resulting in a rupture and subsequent small hole in the back wall of the heart. The tamponade I had diagnosed was caused by bleeding slowly through this rupture into the pericardium. The pressure of the fluid inside the pericardium had effectively been 'sealing' the hole, preventing more direct bleeding into the pericardial sac. Once the fluid (blood) was removed during the tap, the hole had reopened, causing him to suddenly bleed again. It was simply not seen when he was taken back to the operating room as he was not actively bleeding at the time. Once he was moved to the recovery room the hole re-opened and the bleeding into his chest cavity was the point of no return.

It was important for me to have learned that an error or technical mistake during the pericardiocentesis was not the direct cause of his death, per se. Paul's death was due to a complication of the heart attack days earlier, resulting in a small muscular rupture. The diagnosis of tamponade was accurate. I had the knowledge to suspect the diagnosis. I had the skills necessary to both diagnose the problem, and to intervene. Yet it was my failure to have considered this specific cause of his tamponade, my lack of experience, that was a contributor to his death. I had not considered that this recent post-operative heart attack might have caused a rupture, and that this fluid collection might be due to slow bleeding through the hole. I had not seen this during training. I had not 'been there' before. If I had considered it, I would never have tapped the fluid. This rupture could have been fixed with a surgical patch.

The subsequent conversation with the family as to the cause of death was left to the surgeon. It was, after all, his patient. I had only met Paul so briefly. Somehow, that 'distance', not knowing the patient, seems to lessen the impact of their passing. This, again, is part of the emotional survival mechanism I spoke of earlier. But I have never forgotten any of the truly terrible outcomes I have been a part of in my clinical life. With time, and experience, the impact seems to lessen. And not because I don't care. I simply would be unable to function. Paul's passing happened more than thirty years ago, but I remember it in precise detail. I still feel it. I still feel the fear when that code blue was called, and they wheeled him out of ICU to the operating theatre, the chest open. The sickening feeling that accompanies a disaster in the making, one created by you. Complications don't just happen spontaneously. They result from something done by someone. One cannot live, however, nor function, by hanging on to these feelings and thoughts. You learn, you struggle, you move on. You do the best you can do with the tools that you have. Pushing devices inside the heart is no small thing.

Looking back decades later, this is not a mistake I would ever make again. Once again, a bad judgement leading to experience leading to good judgement. This early tug of war between the power of knowledge and the fears due to inexperience would have to remain with me for the time being. I was only months into being a real doctor. It would take a long time for this rivalry of conflicting emotions to become a lasting and stable marriage.

CHAPTER 5
The day-to-day

Life is as tedious as a twice-told tale.

— William Shakespeare

When I was a younger man, a boy really, temporary or part-time jobs littered my life. For most of the jobs that I could be hired for, given my limited experience, I struggled to understand how the 'grown-ups' I worked with managed to work in these settings seemingly forever. How did they tolerate what seemed to me to be nothing more than the same day after day? No excitement. No learning. No adventure. Looking back, of course, the kind of work I could obtain was not necessarily for those building a career path, but merely a means to an end. Making a living until something better came along. Paying the bills of life. My limited experiences, working as a janitor in a shopping mall, a dishwasher, working in an office, doing physical labour on a building site all had one thing in common. The commonplace. The routine. The boring. Outside of any social environment that might be created with others, the routine of work was not one where dreams were built. Well, at least not for me.

My life would be different now, so I told myself. Each and every day would bring new surprises and new excitements. It is one of the wonderful parts of the interventional profession! No consecutive days seem quite the same. You wake up in the morning and often have no idea what may unfold that particular day. It is rare that there is not something, *something*, that will happen that you will learn from. The lessons can be medical or non-medical. An interesting observation, a social patient interaction, a conversation with a colleague. A major emergency. A technical 'victory' in the lab. Maybe watching someone else do something that will add to your repertoire of skills. If you enjoy the learning process, there is much in the world of medical practice to enjoy. But each day can also present itself with yet another new disaster. I like to think that the reader has already seen how fast, how suddenly a smooth day can turn for the worst. This too, has something to teach, but with far less enjoyment associated with it.

But like most things in life, the majority of one's days are eventually anchored in the routine, the ordinary. In the beginning, nothing seemed quite routine. In training, everything was new. The first time I watched an angiogram being done, I thought, *how did he do that?* It almost seemed magical! But with time, like with most jobs, much of the routine can be quite challenging to endure. I suspect this is likely true in all work, all jobs. In particular, I think that when one is providing service to others, the sheer volume of the mundane can become banal and at times, blatantly boring. Laying carpet, painting walls, replacing tires … all tradespeople ultimately see and deal with the same issues over and over again. What is it like to work at the motor vehicles department? How many essays does a high school teacher have to read to see someone with promise? Real estate transactions, traffic violations, last wills and testaments to file ... you get my drift. To someone doing these necessary chores of life, the passage of time can make much of the work a bit of drudgery. Yet, once in a while, a new twist or something of interest occurs that captures one's attention.

Those of us who work as interventionalists are after all, a kind of tradesman, just with a much, much longer education. We have a task at hand to diagnose and maybe to repair, and armed with the tools of the trade, go about our handicraft. The subject matter is, however, not an inanimate object. Not a roof, an automobile, a bicycle, a legal document. It's the living. The breathing. It's personal. About as personal as it gets. Maybe a minor problem, or maybe not. Each case very individually dealt with. The art of practicing medicine. You can learn all you want academically, but the practice of medicine, with patients sitting in front of you, is part evidence-based science, and part art form. With all of this being said, you must excuse me for feeling that there are days that can be quite ... humdrum. Outright not interesting! Never more so than in the office setting.

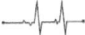

The office of a cardiologist is much like any doctor's office. On any given day, the majority of those walking through the front door have no new problems and are known patients coming for routine follow-up. New patients are referred by other general physicians or specialists for a wide range of reasons. Perhaps an abnormal ECG tracing, a heart murmur, a new physical complaint that may or may not be cardiac, or even a follow-up of a previously known cardiac condition after a long hiatus between visits. In almost all cases the patient is stable. A referral may be made for a medical complaint that is relatively new, within the last week, and the triaging and selection of those patients to be urgently seen must be addressed by either the cardiologist or knowledgeable staff. But by and large, over 90 per cent of patients are fine. Tests may or may not be ordered and prescriptions may be given. For an experienced physician, most of the work is comfortable and relaxed. A good day is filled with interesting cases to assess. Many, many days, however, are filled with common issues seen a thousand times a year.

In the hospital, where patients are acutely ill, there is rarely a sense of boredom. With each clinical presentation, there is something to be diagnosed and if necessary, and if possible, fixed. In the field of cardiology, the real 'action' is in the hospital. It is there where, as a physician, you see the most interesting things along with the most dangerous. Decisions are made quickly in real time. Successful management is measured in days, and sometimes in mere hours. The health and progress of an admitted patient is a very dynamic affair, providing rapid feedback to physicians and testing our ability to adapt and alter our treatment approach. With cardiac interventions, these time frames are further reduced, sometimes to minutes. Outcomes can be measured patient by patient.

The outpatient setting, the office practice, however, is a different matter. Rarely associated with the word 'excitement'. Essential, yes. But exciting, not so much. There is an old Dunkin' Donuts commercial that played in the US, where the hapless donut baker is awakened at 3 a.m. by his alarm. He sits up with his perturbed face and says, 'Time to make the donuts.' Every day, time to make the donuts. Monotony afflicts all walks of life. Medicine is no different.

In the office you see a range of problems and personalities. There is an enormous privilege that comes with my profession. Patients bring with them their trust along with their problems, willing to answer almost anything I am willing to ask. Anything. It's quite a rare relationship. I don't expect that people share what we discuss with the neighbours or the postman. I have tried to honour that relationship. All that I can do to repay that trust is to apply my knowledge and skill to the best of my ability, and hope that such a trade would suffice. Some of the patients became more akin to friends, bringing a smile to my face when I would note that they were due in the office that day. One such patient was responsible for teaching me the basics of fly fishing, an activity generally not learned in the streets of the Bronx, where I grew up. It was a terrific gift. I have received wonderful gifts and goodwill over the years, always hoping that what I could offer in return was enough. If the high-risk end of this profession has made me case-hardened, then the relationships I have developed in the office bring back some of the softness or gentleness that I started out with early in my career. If the hospital is where the tension and buzz reside, it is the office where the relationships evolve.

Some patients, however, can be a different story. I don't mean to be offensive in any way, but just let me say that there are some individuals that can be quite 'challenging' to deal with, even if they may be decent and kind human beings. Understanding the stress that patients can feel in the office is part of the deal, or the art of practice. Nevertheless, it can be a trying experience for all involved, meaning mostly me.

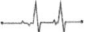

Helen was a woman in her late sixties to early seventies, who had a problem with one of her heart valves. A very common problem associated most often with degeneration and thickening of the valve itself. The problem, *aortic stenosis*, is one in which the valve becomes heavily calcified and simply doesn't open normally, much like the hinges of a rusty door. The typical symptoms of chest discomfort and becoming short of breath were what brought her to the office. The diagnosis was strongly suggested on auscultation of the heart with a stethoscope, and ultimately confirmed with an ultrasound of the heart, called an echocardiogram. So called 'echoes', have been game changers over the past forty years, and have a high degree of accuracy for aortic stenosis with virtually no risk to the patient. Her diagnosis was absolute and straightforward. Left untreated, severe aortic stenosis will inexorably lead to worsening symptoms and, ultimately, to death. Once she was told of the diagnosis, however, the tug of war began. The treatment for this type of valve problem thirty years ago, when she was being seen, was always surgical valve replacement, assuming the patient was fit enough for surgery, which she certainly was. This was not an option she was particularly happy with.

Our next visit brought her to the office with a list of potential diagnostic studies to be done on the heart, to further verify, or refute, the diagnosis. In today's world, it would be obvious that she was a 'victim' of Dr Google. What she needed was to go to the cardiac cath lab to have her coronary vessels assessed and confirm the severity of the valve abnormality. But she had other ideas about this. She clearly had done a lot of homework before seeing me again. Thus, armed with her list, she initiated a lengthy conversation covering every cardiac test known to humankind, which, in her mind, would make it clear that she did not have what I told her she had. I think it is safe to say that most of the conversation was irrelevant. In an era prior to internet capability,

The Day-to-Day

she did, in fact, have an impressive list of tests done for cardiac patients. Unfortunately for her, or maybe for me as well, this list had nothing to add to the diagnosis and was mostly a waste of time. But we learn in this business of providing service to those with critical problems, our patience (as opposed to patients') can be tested, and we must remind ourselves that we are also here to teach and inform. So, teach and inform I dutifully did, and after a prolonged time I convinced her to have her angiogram, and we would then decide whether she would need an operation. (I already knew, of course, that she did.)

She finally was brought to the cath lab for this next study, confirming what the echo had demonstrated, and fortunately for her there were no problems with the coronary arteries. The definitive treatment was a surgical valve replacement. This was as straightforward a case as anyone could ask. Low-risk surgery. Typically, great result. Relief of symptoms and prolongation of life. What else can you ask for when you walk in with a life-threatening problem?

Upon our next office follow-up, she was now armed with an article in the *US News and World Report*, an American magazine rated as a top source of news. This article – she had brought me a copy – listed the top fifteen or so American cardiac centres where valve surgery was performed, giving all the reasons to fly there for one's surgery. I personally have no problem with a patient going wherever they wish to, if it eases their mind. But I also made it clear that valve surgery was low risk, highly successful, and done by virtually every cardiac surgeon in any cardiac centre in the world. This was not some specialized operation akin to heart transplant, which is restricted to those centres with the necessary support structures in place. This was not a congenital abnormality rarely seen in adults that required a surgeon specializing in the field. Valve operations are done almost daily, almost everywhere. Again, if she wished to go fly to another city to have it done, it would be fine by me. But I felt an obligation to tell her she was in good hands where we lived, and there truly was no good reason to go elsewhere. It was important for her to also understand that you simply don't walk out of the hospital after surgery and jump back on a plane and go home. There is significant time in cardiac rehabilitation, alongside surgical follow-up which must be considered as part of the whole journey. And so this conversation, with the magazine opened in front of me (including the litany of testing services offered, again), continued until finally she accepted surgery locally. These conversations felt as if I'd had to arm wrestle her to the ground. But at least I knew I was providing her with due diligence.

She had her surgery. Everything went fine and within five days she was discharged. No complications. A typically good outcome for this type of valve replacement.

Approximately a week later she called my nurse in the office, complaining of constipation. Yes, constipation. After all the time I had spent with her, with all the explanations of this and that, after finally getting her to acquiesce to the right corrective treatment, the last thing on this planet I was interested in was her constipation! I know it was important to her, but you must remember I was not a general family doctor. This was a 'clinical' issue that I was not particularly interested in managing. If she couldn't breathe properly, if she had pain in her chest, if she had leg swelling, if she had any number of post-operative problems that may be due to the cardiovascular system, I was getting involved. But constipation? Anyway, I said to my nurse to tell her, 'We don't do constipation – call your general physician.' And with those simple words, she was insulted enough, felt the care was not good enough, never to return to the practice again.

After all that had transpired with the wrestling and the magazines, and the articles and the testing, it all came down to being constipated. Don't get me wrong. When this kind of thing happens, one is quietly relieved that further conversations will likely never take place again. But it certainly reminds you, some patients do fit the category of 'challenging'.

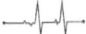

And yet, others can be so delightful. If not always exciting, the office can give you a chance to really get to know people over time. I have learned so much about so many things having nothing to do with medicine. I have learned about excavators, bee keeping, potato farming. I have learned about soil content and fertilizers, plumbing, electricity, glider planes … all from tradespeople and amateurs. The old and the young. Those gracious enough to answer silly questions I have about topics so seemingly simple to them, but new horizons for me. I have spent the better part of my life in the world of academics and medicine.

I grew up on the concrete streets of the Bronx. I could not fathom why someone, one day, drove past me on the street, stopped, and asked me if I had seen a swarm of bees fly past, as she raced to catch them. *WHAT?!!!* That was my reaction. Who runs towards a swarm of bees! From where I come from, it is pretty low on the list of things to chase. Don't you run in the opposite direction? She *wants* a swarm of bees? Well, now I know why. Took a few years, but one day a patient brought me a tub of his home-made honey, and I learned about bees. And if you don't know anything about this, you can look it up and read about it. It's interesting stuff and now I know a lot more about bees, knowledge absolutely worth knowing.

I have had patients bring me gifts over the years. I am always touched by their good thoughts and generosity. I have never thought that after an office visit, anyone would think of me. Why would they? I am but a small player in their worlds. And yet, when a gift is given, I realize that to get this token, they had to have thought of me. And wanted to show appreciation. It is rather touching. Liquor has been common – and put to good use! (Spoiler: I am not a big drinker but happy to share with friends and family.) I have received fresh fish caught in local waters, Scotch brought back from Scotland specifically for me, honey collected from personal hives, books penned by my patients, a hand-crafted knife with images of the local geography carved on the handle, fresh eggs right from the hen. One patient compiled a short story book written by her six children, thanking me for giving them back their mom. And perhaps one for the ages, a lead-glass-blown clock in the image of an anatomic heart, accompanied by a note simply saying 'Thanks for giving me time'. Wow. To say that I am touched by these gifts fails to do justice to the acts. They have helped sustain me through many disillusioned moments.

And while the office has its ups and downs, once in a while you are truly brought to attention. One day, William, an 80-year-old, fairly fit man, came into the office just having driven himself from home approximately half an hour away. William walked in, took off his coat, hung his hat on the rack and, in the middle of the waiting room, had a sudden cardiac arrest. This, in a waiting room full of people. No pulse, no blood pressure. We began CPR. The defibrillator was brought out, and he was shocked back into life.

This, in a time era when defibrillators were not readily found in the community as they are often now. In those days, defibrillators were to be found in hospitals, and, if the right kind of doctor, in their office. This being a cardiac practice, such a device was kept on site, although almost never used. But here we were, defibrillating a patient back to life in the waiting room of the office. Can you imagine those sitting in the waiting room seeing this happen? We called an ambulance, and he was transferred fairly quickly to the hospital. The ECG showed he was having a heart attack, and he was brought quickly to the cardiac cath lab for an emergency intervention. I discovered the problem and was fortunately able to fix it with a balloon (before stents were available), and William walked out of the hospital alive. A month later he was back in the office with no problems. The crisis was instantaneous, the cure fast and timely. This is again an example of the nature of the beast, so to speak.

Years later, at the end of another routine office day seeing follow-ups and refilling prescriptions, a gentleman in his fifties showed up with profound and progressive breathlessness. He could barely get into the office. I saw him with no clue what was happening, but he was definitely not well. When he went out to the secretary, he almost collapsed. He had no chest pain, but he was feeling terrible. He was not someone with chronic health issues; this clearly was not normal for him. He had a history of previous cardiac disease, and thus I sent him straight to the hospital by ambulance. His wife was with him, but he was so ill-appearing I felt that an ambulance was required. Later that same day, having finished with the outpatient list, I returned to the hospital, something I would not normally have needed to do that day. I brought him urgently to the cath lab and discovered critical pathology, again, fixable with stenting. He walked out of the hospital within 24 hours, and three months later he was back in the office for routine follow-up as if nothing had ever been wrong with him.

I have told this old joke many a time:

Q. What does the doctor do when the patient is leaving his office and drops dead as he is stepping out the door?
A. Turns him around and makes it look as if he's walking in!

It's a timeless joke and always gets a laugh from the right audience. Picking the 'right' audience is part of the art of practice, rather than the science. But I have also been lucky. There have been a few close calls, but I have never had to 'turn them around'. Much of the time, the office is akin to the baker awakening at 3 a.m. saying 'Time to make the donuts' … But every now and then, there are some *great* donuts to be made.

CHAPTER 6
The cath lab

Teamwork is the fuel that allows common people to attain uncommon results.

— Andrew Carnegie

It is a fact that despite spending years honing skills in the cath lab, an interventionalist spends most of their time doing 'non-interventional' things. When fellows leave the world of training, where you operate daily, and start the life of a consultant, it can come as a shock of sorts to find out you are not in the cath lab every day. Unless you have the type of practice where patients are being sent to you only for your technical skill, your 'hands', so to speak, most time is spent talking to patients and doing the day-to-day clinical work required to attend to any number of clinical problems. But where most interventionalists really want to be is the cath lab. Virtually every story in these writings takes place there. For this is the place where cardiac catheterization is done. The room where the detailed truth of coronary anatomy is discovered. Where intracardiac tools are utilized, measuring parameters that accurately reflect cardiac structure and function. The place where life and death can be witnessed in mere moments. Where lifesaving manoeuvres are performed if you are good enough and trained well enough to do the work. This is where the action is. This is where the operator has the greatest impact. Confronted with both elective and emergency problems, the skills obtained through many years of training are put to use. In the minds of some young trainees, this is, maybe, where they can be a hero.

In chapter 1, I alluded to the curious use of the term 'procedure' to describe what is done in the cath lab. For me, the use of this word miserably fails to do justice to the risks and benefits of the work that is done. A mole removal, a tooth extraction, ear wax removal – these are procedures. A hernia repair is an operation. Tonsillectomy ... an operation. Guiding catheters, wires, balloons and such through the circulation inside the blood vessels of the heart and then inflating devices in territory with life altering consequence ... a procedure. I know ... it's just words.

Similarly, the term 'lab' is an interesting one, connotating a place of experimentation, with bubbling beakers and Bunsen burners. These words profoundly downplay the activities that take place in this room. I would venture to say, despite my bias, that day to day, the risks encountered in the 'lab' are far greater than anywhere else in the hospital building. It is a very specialized and unique environment. Take a physician or surgeon or nurse or anyone trained in any aspect of medical practice, no matter how experienced, and in this room, they will be lost. It is unlike any space that operates on patients. This is the place, the room, where I have spent my professional life.

While the basics of the procedures done in the cath lab have been around for decades, the diagnostic tools used have dramatically evolved, along with everything else. Smaller tools have allowed us to make smaller 'holes' in order to gain vascular access, making bleeding complications less likely. The 'catheters' that we use to access the heart have significantly evolved, with a myriad of shapes and sizes to accommodate almost anyone's anatomy with less physical manipulation. The goal of this progress has been to make all invasive work simpler, quicker, and less risky. Yet I remember, during my training, having an electric hot plate in the back of the room whose purpose was to boil sterile saline, so that we could place catheters in the hot saline and literally bend them into different shapes to fit the anatomy of the patient. To suggest that to a trainee today would only result in a bewildered stare.

The very idea that you could thread hollow plastic tubing (polyurethane, polyethylene), which is a perhaps an oversimplification of a catheter, through the body, into the heart and manage not to do serious damage along the way is astonishing. And that it can be done without anyone dying in the process. A century ago, in 1929, Werner Forssman, a German resident hoping to practice cardiology, numbed up his own arm and threaded a urinary catheter via the antecubital vein into the right atrium of his heart. It had never been done: it was thought that to put a device inside the heart would lead to death. This 'insane' manoeuvre was done without permission of the hospital. He went on to record the images of the catheter with a plain chest x-ray, proving that placing an external device, such as a catheter, inside a beating heart would not cause sudden death. The famous photograph of Forssman sitting with the catheter in his arm was taken by a nurse, documenting that he had performed it on himself (one can google the image). Since the procedure had not been given clearance by the hospital that employed him, he subsequently lost his position there, ultimately finding work elsewhere. His reputation preceded him in those early years, and he gave up on cardiology and entered training in urology. His life would have been left in obscurity but for the work years later by two cardiologists in the US, who would take his work much further to study intracardiac flow dynamics. In 1956, Forssman would return from the 'wilderness' of medicine and share the Nobel Prize in Physiology or Medicine with André Cournand and Dickinson Richards for their work in advancing the field of cardiac investigations.

While it was then accepted that one could place catheters inside the heart without risking death, in the early 1950s it was still believed that if you injected the iodinated contrast dye (the dye that is still currently used to visualise the artery) into the coronary vessels, you would die. Catheters, at that time, were being used to measure pressures within the various heart chambers and to inject dye into the aorta or left ventricle. Most of this work was performed to investigate various forms of congenital heart disease or adult valvular heart disease. The first coronary angiogram was ultimately performed in 1958 at the Cleveland Clinic by Dr Mason Sones. It was an accident. Dr Sones was a paediatric cardiologist who was performing a catheterization on a 26-year-old patient with rheumatic valvular heart disease. In this case, what was to be another seminal moment in cardiology, the contrast was injected into the root of the ascending aorta, when by sheer accident, the catheter slipped into the right coronary artery, resulting in the vessel filling with contrast. Upon seeing this was happening in real time, Sones jumped up to the table with scalpel in hand and was immediately preparing to open the patient's chest to perform internal heart compression. And yet … nothing happened. The patient survived. And as simple as that, the advent of invasive coronary angiography happened. The result of an accident. Coronary angiography would evolve in time, but the word 'procedure' never seemed to disappear. A hernia repair: an operation. Manipulation of intracardiac devices: a procedure.

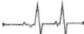

The cath lab is where this all happens. To the eyes of most, it is not unlike a standard operating theatre, but there are some major differences. The air circulation is different, as the risk of wound infection is far greater in a standard operating room, given the size of the surgical openings created. We 'puncture' blood vessels with small needles: the likelihood of infection is quite low. There are differences in the anaesthetic equipment as well, since in the cath lab, anaesthesia is rarely used except for in an emergency. Unlike most surgical theatres, the cath lab works with x-ray equipment. The x-rays serve as our eyes into the chest. Without functioning x-rays, we simply cannot see the anatomy. We are blind. Thus, radiation safety needs be maintained, including lead shielding throughout the walls.

Radiation safety is a significant concern. To the patients, yes. To those who work there daily, very much so. The exposure time to radiation is extremely variable, case to case, and lead aprons are worn by all staff who work in the room during the duration of each procedure, covering most of the body as well as the neck, with the thyroid gland particularly sensitive to radiation exposure. These lead aprons are then covered by the surgical scrub gowns, so are not always seen by the patients. The weight of the lead apron is quite variable and as with all things, has improved with time. Nevertheless, the weight of the apron cannot be reduced to nothing, for nothing gives you no protection. When nurses and trainees first come to work in the lab, the end of the day may find them quite fatigued due to the sheer weight of wearing these things all day long. You get accustomed to it with time, and it is not something you think about. But many a time I remember scrubbing in on a case thinking how good and strong I felt, only to discover that I simply forgot to put the 'lead' on! What a difference to wear a gown with no lead. You feel so light.

Scrubbing to be at the table never gets old if you love this stuff. There is that mix of excitement and fear early in one's career. (Actually, I am pretty certain that it never completely disappears.) You simply don't know what you are going to come across. Every person has somewhat different anatomy. While there are often very routine cases, where no difficulty is encountered, it is amazing to see how often an operator gets 'stuck', having a slight hiccup that has to be worked around to finish the case. Fortunately, the gear we use is so very reliable and predictable that getting 'stuck' becomes less frequent with time and experience. And thank goodness, so does the fear factor. It subsides with time, lingering in the background of thought.

At the table is the primary operator, usually the consultant, who virtually always has a nurse scrubbed in with them to assist handling the equipment. In teaching hospitals, there is usually a trainee or fellow working alongside the consultant, also scrubbed in for the case. As the trainee gains experience, they may be moved to the head of the table and become the primary operator with the consultant alongside. In the room is a circulating nurse, there to get additional gear you may need and to administer drugs to the patient. Their primary role is to be there for the patient and watch over them. This includes medication that may be routine, as well as drugs that may be required when things are not going according to plan. The circulating nurse plays a critical role despite not being at the table. Keeping an eye on the patient (remember, they are awake) and watching over all things in the room, while those at the table are focused on the 'action' that is taking place inside the patient's chest and seen on the viewing screen. When things do go south, the circulating nurse may be called upon to do ten things at once. It is a vital role and not to be left to those with little knowledge or experience. When circulating nurses are in training, they are always accompanied by one more senior to step in when things get a bit crazy.

Along with those in the room, who are wearing lead, there is a nurse who is watching all the monitors and tracings of the heart from the next room, the control room, which is separated from the inner lab by lead glass. They see all that is happening, adding extra eyes to all vital signs, ECG tracings, and heart rhythms. They are often the first to see when life-threatening electrical problems occur and are expected to let everyone in the room know. They must be prepared to crash into the room to assist in an arrest.

The team is rounded out by the radiographer, whose job it is to keep an eye on the x-ray and imaging equipment. The imaging equipment has come a very long way over the past decades. The videos taken now are all digital and can be reviewed immediately. Years ago, images were obtained on film, thus requiring the radiographer to grab the film canister at the end of the case and bring it to the developing room before images could be reviewed. Digital imaging has been instrumental in making cases go smoother and quicker, allowing decisions to be made almost instantaneously. Today's imaging equipment also has numerous modalities of use, and the radiographer's job is to know how to use them all. If you are really lucky, as I have been, your chief radiographer will be intimately familiar with all the various imaging modalities. And if you are even luckier, they will be far more than a technician, but someone who you can rely on to troubleshoot all kinds of nonclinical issues that arise in the room. There is an array of equipment that is routinely used outside of x-rays, often a mystery to many who work there. The really good radiographers will be that guy you turn to, to fix that which will not work. When you are in the middle of a case, this is a very, very big thing.

At the top of this pyramid, of course, is the primary operator. Truth being told, they're responsible for everything that happens in that room. Doesn't matter if they don't know how to fix something, or what to do to get around a hiccup. Doesn't matter if the nurse did something wrong, the monitoring nurse didn't see something on the monitor, the fellow or trainee made a foolish or clumsy error. The primary is the primary and is the one responsible. I have loved the role. If the primary operator is good, they are able to do the primary technical work while simultaneously watching that everyone else is doing their jobs. It requires thinking about all things, even when only doing one thing. The needs of the awake patient must always be remembered, even when engrossed in some particularly complex technical manoeuvre.

Many a day I have finished a case and thought that if a bomb had exploded outside in the hallway, I would never even have noticed it. You become so engaged, at times, that all else ceases to be. One moment all is running smoothly. The next all hell breaks loose. The patient is awake, sometimes quite ill. Lots of moving parts. Lots of needs to attend to simultaneously. Staff moving quickly, waiting for instructions, the good ones sometimes knowing what to do before the operator has a chance to contemplate it all. When things go south, it's a team effort. The primary operator is in the centre of the circus, but without the team … I wish them well.

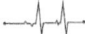

It was approximately midnight on a Saturday when I was called in to see a man in his forties, sent from another hospital, with evidence of an evolving heart attack. By the majority of worldwide standards, it was a fairly late presentation of his problem, evolving over the previous 12 hours. The ECG was diagnostic, and he was clinically stable.

Let me briefly talk about what constitutes a 'late' presentation before I go on. Generally, after a certain number of hours have passed, even opening up blocked arteries may not be of great significance to the patient. The damage to heart muscle may be complete. It's the equivalent of closing the barn door after the horse has bolted. During an acute heart attack, the reason we open up blocked blood vessels is to preserve cardiac function. That is why time is of the essence. If late in the evolution of a heart attack, you may end up with an open artery, but perhaps too late. The damage is complete and thus the heart muscle tissue has died. Imagine taking a severed finger to the emergency department 48 hours after it was cut off. The likelihood of reattachment and return of function is virtually non-existent. The same can be true with heart muscle. Re-establishing blood flow to an area already damaged may simply be more cosmetic than functional. As we say during a heart attack, time is muscle.

However, it's not always easy to be certain when 'late' is 'too late'. And often when we encounter these types of late presentations, particularly in young individuals with long life expectancies, we will lean in the direction of an aggressive approach. The threshold to take a young patient having an acute cardiac event to the lab is low.

So, in the early morning hours, this young gentleman was taken to the lab after the team was called in. It was found that one major artery (the left anterior descending artery or LAD) was acutely blocked, being the cause of his heart attack. A second major vessel (the right coronary artery or RCA) was also found to be totally blocked, but by its appearance, clearly for a long time (these are referred to as chronic total occlusions). There is only one other major vessel in the heart (the left circumflex artery or LCx), which was fortunately normal, and obviously the reason he was still alive. Anatomically, in this young man, the normal artery and the acutely blocked vessel came off a common trunk, called the left main artery, which in this case was highly pertinent. That night, the goal was to simply re-establish flow in the 'culprit' acutely occluded vessel (the LAD) and go home. Not always simple but at least 'straightforward', the word I had, by then, learned was highly suspect!

The catheters were switched for the appropriate equipment to be deployed and off we went. No sooner did I place the second catheter in his heart than his left main artery became torn or *dissected*. And there was no flow. So, let me summarize this situation. Pay attention. What I am describing is that he has one acutely blocked artery, one chronically blocked artery, and now the only remaining normal artery, which was keeping him alive, is completely dissected with zero flow. There is no flow to his heart, anywhere. That is correct. He has no blood supply to his heart. With no flow, no blood supply to the heart, this motor, this engine, will cease to work.

When I saw this dissection, I remember standing there almost without emotion, thinking *This man is about to die.* You cannot survive when all vessels in the heart are gone. I recall a certain calm descending over me. A strange sensation given what was about to transpire. I have read that drowning victims, before they lose consciousness, have a feeling of calmness, relaxation and peace. I don't know if that is true or not, but I do know that it is akin to what I was feeling at that moment. I was very aware that it was not my life slipping away. It was the inevitability of this young man's passing. It is quite a sight when there is no flow to any portion of the heart! Nothing! But I had a secret weapon at my disposal. I had my team. I knew what to do. And so did they. It was to be a thing of beauty.

A code is immediately called, and a team of outside help crashes into the room. I suspect we have maybe 30 to 60 seconds at most before he is gone. While I'm calling out for the equipment I hope to use to repair the damage I have done with my catheter, the other vascular access point (the left femoral artery) is being prepped and draped, with preparation for an intra-aortic balloon pump if needed. I am watching the patient, who is now looking around the room wondering what the commotion is all about. I know what the commotion is about. He is still conscious at that point but very, very soon he will not be. There's no time to talk to him. And what could one say in moments like this? Meanwhile, our monitoring nurse has left the control room and is sliding under the table at lightning speed, hooking up all the necessary cables and attachments for the equipment about to be deployed. This young man's heart rate is gradually slowing and is about to go flat line. Patients often begin to have seizure-like activity at this point and must be guarded against falling off the table or accidentally dislodging equipment inside their heart. A complex and life-threatening scenario can get even more complicated if you are not careful! Once unconscious, which occurs rather quickly, he is then intubated and ventilated.

My scrub nurse already knows what I will need and is running around the room prepping the emergency equipment. With the scrub nurse preoccupied, the circulating nurse is assisting the code team. (Even the radiographers will put on lead and jump into the room to get the equipment I am asking for, despite this not being their primary role.)

Meanwhile, within less than 30 seconds, I manage to slide a small wire through the dissection site and, with a little skill and a lot of luck, end up in the right place. I use a balloon to open what was once a normal vessel and within a minute I've deployed a stent. Flow to the dissected artery is restored gradually. And now his heart is returning to a normal rhythm and his BP is gradually climbing. The balloon pump is put in and after another half hour I have managed to open the acutely occluded blood vessel that brought us there to begin with.

The patient is moved to the ICU. He is stable, with excellent blood pressure, normal heart rhythm, and ventilated with the aid of a machine. The lab room is a mess. Equipment all over the room. Tidy working conditions were not the priority in this case! Speed and efficiency was the name of the game. It's two o'clock in the morning, and the team is cleaning up.

I write my notes and dictate the report. We have dodged a huge bullet this time. It is nuts. The patient arrived awake and alert, only to be moments away from death with the slight manipulation of a coronary catheter. The staff and I can only look at one another, here, in the middle of the night, and nod our heads knowing what we have witnessed. We nearly ended this man's life in the attempt to make him better. Yet we got him through it. Yes, we. This was not just me. It was us. That young man will walk out of the building five days later with no recollection of what transpired.

This is the cath lab. This is the team. This is where the action is. This is where 'procedures' are done.

CHAPTER 7
So long ago

The world breaks everyone and afterward many are strong at the broken places.

— Ernest Hemingway

With a year or two now under my belt, I was beginning to feel … comfortable. I continued to adapt to the rhythm of the workday, starting with patient rounds in the hospital, seeing new patients as well as those who needed follow up visits.

If you are a solo practitioner that means you are the one rounding daily. It's a smaller number of patients to see, but nevertheless, always the beginning of your workday. But most cardiology practices are now group practices, and thus the responsibility of inpatient care rotates on a schedule set by the group. Priority in the order of patients being seen is based on the nature of the problem. The requests for consults can be anything from a simple check on a previous patient of the practice, to patients with new cardiac complaints. The questions and thinking are not much different to those of the outpatient setting; the major difference is the level of acuity of illness. This, and the rather obvious fact that the patients are in a bed, wearing little but a hospital gown, often with an intravenous cannula inserted somewhere in their arm. It is fascinating how different people appear when in a hospital bed versus wearing their normal daily clothing. Seen in the hospital, dressed in the less-than-fashionable standard wardrobe, people look sicker even when they are well. Seen in the office, wearing normal clothing, they may appear quite well, even when they are not. What a surprise, and a delightful one at that, to meet someone for the first time in the office after they have left hospital, no longer wearing the official hospital attire! You can almost believe they are cured.

For the past few decades, time and efficiency have been key components in the management of hospitalized patients, given the costs involved in keeping people in a hospital bed. Being efficient with the management of someone ill, while avoiding premature hospital discharge, has been one of the greatest challenges clinicians have faced in the economics of modern-day health care. Premature discharges are known to lead to early readmissions, so are to be avoided. Yet the pressure to move patients through the admission and discharge process has been driven both by the need for the bed to be vacated for others and, not to be discounted, the economics of health care. How hospitals are paid and how much money is collected from insurers is a significant factor in health care delivery. These drivers of discharging patients, the need for beds and the funding of hospitals, are quite different from country to country given the different health care reimbursement programs in place. While the economics of health care is clearly beyond the scope of this book, it deserves mention given its impact on how long people remain in the building and how quickly and efficiently management is carried out.

Exact times and years have escaped me as I write these stories retrospectively. But there are 'eras' that allow me to place my memories into blocs of time. As noted, my earliest cases were done prior to the advent and utilization of cardiac stents. In that earlier time, vessels were opened with a balloon with the hope that the vessel would simply remain open. But the mechanical trauma that the balloon creates to the wall of the artery can cause great harm to the inner lining of the vessel, leading to a tear in the wall, known as dissection.

An artery has multiple 'layers' in its wall, each layer providing certain physical properties to that artery. The inner layer, the *intima*, is the thinnest. Deeper in the artery is the muscular and elastic layer, followed by a third layer which is basically fibrous tissue that holds it all together, known as *adventitia*. A dissected or torn artery can be visualized akin to a thin layer of wallpaper being peeled off the underlying wall. The inner layer, or intima, develops a slight tear that allows it to separate from the second, or muscular layer of the vessel, just like peeling wallpaper. Next, imagine that water is now running behind this torn piece of wallpaper, tracking down the wall further, causing more wallpaper to be lifted up. This is what occurs with a dissected artery. But it's not water flowing behind that slight tear; it's blood. Since the blood flowing in the artery now can enter this 'torn' spot, it may track between the inner lining and the second or muscular layer, causing it to peel or lift off the underlying wall. This 'dissection plane' may be limited in size, if the tear is small, or, when the tear is bigger, very, very large. To take this even one step further, in the most extreme instances, the balloon may not only tear the inner layer but perforate a hole through all three layers of the vessel, through the intima, muscular layer and outer adventitial layer. Such a 'rupture' of the full thickness of the vessel wall leads to acute bleeding, with blood exiting the artery and flowing into the pericardium. Depending on the size of the perforation in the vessel, patients can become rather acutely ill, and in worst-case scenarios, potentially die. Quickly.

These problems, a dissection or perforation, can be the consequence of opening up a diseased artery simply by the inflation of a balloon. Why not choose a smaller balloon or perhaps not inflate it so much, you might ask? If not ballooned aggressively enough, the vessel might merely stretch, only to recoil to its original diseased size. Too large, with pressures too great, can lead to major vessel trauma. Both ends of the spectrum fail to result in a good outcome for the person lying on the table. It was a tricky balancing act. Being aggressive enough to obtain a good and long-lasting result, against the risk of creating a much larger problem.

Stenting was a game changer. The metallic stent, originally made with stainless steel, acted to seal any tear or dissection created by the inflation of a balloon. If the underlining wall was torn, the presence of this metal scaffold would literally tack up the flap (like gluing up the torn wallpaper). Additionally, given the structural integrity, or strength, of this scaffold, it would prevent recoil of the vessel. Stents had their own problems associated with them, but when the stent 'era' arrived, coronary interventions were forever changed. The failure rate of angioplasty dramatically diminished. With a nice result, that is, the target artery now at its normal size with the stent fully deployed, one could more comfortably leave the cath lab knowing that the acute complications that had been routine were significantly lessened. When I began, one would see a patient leave the cath lab for emergency open heart surgery nearly once every couple of weeks. Yet now, the need for emergency bypass surgery is a rarity. A busy cath lab may have years go by without any surgical emergency interventions.

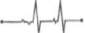

A 58-year-old gentleman was undergoing a balloon dilatation of a coronary vessel for unstable angina. Once positioned, the balloon was expanded, deflated, and boom, a large dissection ensued. One inflation was all it took. But not only did the vessel wall tear or dissect, it dissected in a very 'ugly' way. This type of the dissection is called a spiral. Rather than just a localized, linear, straight-line tear (the most common appearance), this dissection type extended over a long distance of the vessel wall, spiralling around all sides of the artery, giving the appearance of barber-pole stripes when contrast dye was injected. As blood, and thus the contrast dye, enters into this false channel behind the torn wall, differentiation of the true from the false channel can be impossible to delineate. Essentially, you cannot tell the difference between where the blood should be flowing, the true channel or lumen, and where the 'false' channel begins and ends. Fixing this type of tear can be a nightmare. Even in today's world, with better imaging and more advanced tools, fixing this kind of dissection can be technically challenging. One will often fail or, if not careful, make it far worse with additional manipulation. Decades ago, when this event occurred, attempting a repair was a fool's folly.

For whatever reason, at least on that day, good fortune was on my side. Despite my 'what am I going to do now' moment, tinged with a sprinkling of anxiety, the patient had absolutely no symptoms. Even with this vessel trauma, torn and spiralled, he felt fine. Many patients in such a situation will suffer severe chest pain alongside ECG changes consistent with an evolving heart attack. But not that day. I watched him for a while, keeping him on the table, simply observing. And nothing was happening. You wait and wait. Waiting for the crash. Anticipating the worst. Preparing yourself for the 'what am I gonna do' next move. But after about a half an hour, I elected to walk away, stop the proceedings, and cross my fingers that all would remain well. As that day progressed, I nervously awaited the call from the ward that he was having troubles. I had already been down this path before, phone calls from nurses letting me know an angioplasty patient from earlier in the day was now having severe chest pain. And yet, I heard nothing. A few days later, with the patient having no symptoms whatsoever, I elected to study him again to see what was happening, what the vessel looked like. And lo and behold, the vessel looked absolutely normal! The dissection had healed, and the site of the angioplasty looked terrific. It had been a successful procedure after all, and despite an anatomic complication, all had healed. Yes, these torn segments can repair without any help from us. And he was back to normal.

Sometimes watchful waiting is the best thing to do. And not for the first time was I to learn that some days it just seems that you are better off being lucky than good. I wish I could say that it always turns out that way.

One of my colleagues was performing a balloon inflation on a critically diseased and calcified blood vessel on a woman in her eighties. Calcification of arteries is due to the build-up of calcium in blood vessels, the result of micro injuries to the arterial wall over many years of living. It becomes more common as we age and can pose different challenges in attempting to fix them with something as simple as balloon pressure. The vessels become physically hard, akin to becoming more like concrete than the very soft and pliable arteries we are born with. This pathology was first described in postmortem examinations dating back to the mid-1800s and was commonly referred to as 'hardening of the arteries', a term that seems to have slowly disappeared from our language. But, in fact, it's a good descriptor of what can occur to blood vessels. They become 'hard' to the touch. And as they harden, you might imagine that it takes more balloon pressure to open the artery. So following balloon inflation, I watched the balloon deflate, to be followed by injection of contrast dye to see if the artery was in fact opened. What I witnessed looked like a 'mushroom cloud' explosion of contrast appearing at the inflation site, indicative of a major perforation in the artery. It all happened so fast, in the literal blink of an eye. It was a shock to see this massive exit of contrast dye outside of the vessel itself! I can still see it. Death would ensue if this was not managed in less than 60 seconds. My colleague was smart enough to put the balloon back into the artery and inflate it, trying to temporarily seal the hole with the inflated balloon while the surgeons were called. Drains needed to be placed into the pericardium to remove the blood that had already been released through the perforation. Within 45 minutes, the patient was having emergency open heart surgery to seal the hole in her artery. She survived.

Complications in this business are commonplace, unpredictable, sudden … and often, unnerving. In this subspecialty, where technical obstacles and complications come frequently, without predictability, losing courage and confidence is a danger to both doctor and patient. No one wants to see a major adverse problem being created. Yet it seems to remain an inevitability in medical practice of all kinds, and having the skills to get through it, repair it, and create a good outcome does contribute to one's sense of professional excellence. There is a particular 'high' that comes with being able to cope when faced with a major complication.

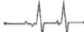

Stanley was a 42-year-old man with fairly typical angina. Coronary angiography demonstrated one artery with a tight blockage, amenable to angioplasty, with a second artery that was completely occluded. How long this total occlusion had been present was unclear. It may have been months or even years. There was no way to be certain. But the 'culprit' problem was clearly the other vessel. We often use that term, culprit, to identify the primary cause of the problem at that time. There may be other issues to deal with, but when approaching a clinical anatomic problem, identifying the 'culprit' allows us greater clarity on how to proceed further. Stanley's culprit was easy to see. The second artery that was totally blocked was not what put him in the hospital. The third major artery was normal, and in my mind, the thing to do was to fix the culprit problem. And so, I went about doing just that, which was smooth and simple. But then I had other ideas. I elected to turn my attention to the totally occluded vessel, thinking, why not give it a shot? What was there to lose (words to always be wary of) as it was already a hundred per cent blocked off? I couldn't make it two hundred per cent! How long it had been that way was unclear to me, but with a patient aged 42, I thought that trying to achieve a complete 'fix' would be a superior option.

I began the usual probing of the vessel with specialized wires to see if I could find the true pathway through this totally occluded vessel. I had no intention of prolonging the procedure needlessly, since I was confident that the clinical problem, the culprit, was fixed and that this second artery was an incidental finding, even if I deemed it to be an important one. After trying for about twenty minutes, and achieving no forward progress, I thought it was not relevant enough, or important enough that day, to persist. I told Stanley it was time to walk away with a good result and consider if anything further should be done in the months ahead. He was then taken off the table, moved to the recovery room, and the next patient was brought in. I was quite happy and content with the outcome.

While I was busy with this next patient, the nurse kept poking her head in the door to tell me that Stanley's blood pressure was down, and he didn't look 'right'. In the middle of another case, I could hardly drop the tools and take a look for myself. But I was moving quickly due to my obvious concerns as to what might be happening.

Once I had finished, I went into the recovery room to have a look. Stanley was quite lethargic, and his BP was running low for him, in the 80/60 range. He was awake, with no specific complaints to relate to me, but there was no question that his affect and personality had changed. Something was not right. I had my suspicions, but it was clear to me that I had to put him back on the table and repeat the angiogram to figure out what was happening. While I was reintroducing the gear, that we had just removed, back into his heart, a cardiac ultrasound was also being done as part of the total evaluation. To make a long story short, I discovered that while trying to open that completely blocked artery, probing around with an assortment of wires, I had perforated the vessel at its occlusion site, and it was slowly bleeding into the pericardium, creating the scenario of cardiac tamponade. The other artery, the culprit, that had been successfully stented, looked fine and was not contributing to the clinical problem at hand. So now, I suppose I had a new culprit. One that I created. Now I had to fix the perforation, again, that I had created, and drain the blood from the pericardium. Watchful waiting was not the answer to this one.

I had never fixed this type of perforation before. I had never even seen one fixed before. This was uncharted territory for me. But like many more cases to come in my life, I had mentally prepared and practiced for such an event. And I had the necessary equipment in the cath lab available to do the work. I had ordered the right 'tools' just in case this were to happen someday. What followed was the deployment of what are referred to as 'vascular coils' into the artery. These are small pieces of an expandable metallic alloy with feather-like projections, which when properly delivered, coil like a Slinky when inserted inside a blood vessel. The feather-like projections are designed to create a blood clot immediately, in order to seal any perforation. I had neither done a coiling procedure, nor seen one done before, but I understood the theory. Were there instructions on the box? That would help. Nope, no instructions. Google it! YouTube? Nothing. It was up to us to figure it out. Vascular coils were not commonly used back then and have gradually become more sophisticated and easier to use. And yes, now there are YouTube videos as well. The scrub nurse and I opened the equipment and worked out step by step how to deliver the coils to the perforation site. After draining the pericardial blood and deploying two coils, the hole was sealed! Stanley's blood pressure returned to baseline almost immediately, and he would walk out of the hospital 36 hours later!

An unnerving complication, to be followed by a fist-pumping successful intervention, fixing the problem that I had created. (Yeah, I did a fist pump.) These are satisfying moments, to be sure, even while you know a catastrophe was in the making. It is the push-pull of this kind of work that makes you run away or keeps you coming back for more.

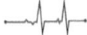

It was earlier, much earlier in my career, when I was asked to see a man in his late forties who had presented with typical angina and ECG changes. I'll call him Mark (not his real name). His past history was otherwise quite unremarkable save for some allergic hay fever. All that was required was an angiogram to establish the anatomic pathology. On the basis of anatomy, a decision was then made for the best course of management. He was discovered to have, yet again, ideal anatomy for angioplasty. Single vessel disease was found in a major artery with the degree of obstruction in the neighbourhood of 95 per cent. Other vessels were pristine, with excellent cardiac function. The decision to proceed with a coronary intervention was quite clear for single vessel pathology. The appropriate option was balloon angioplasty. Despite my earlier complications, I was still young and foolish enough to believe that that which looks straightforward, will thus be so. How many times have I had to learn this lesson!

A wire was used to gain access to the artery. And with one balloon inflation, everything changed. One moment Mark and I were speaking to one another. The next – how quickly all of this transpires. Within seconds, he arrested on the table.

I quickly deflate the balloon and remove it from the artery. There is, yet again, no blood flow through the vessel. A look for clues as to dissection, rupture, clot: Nothing. I conduct prolonged balloon inflations up and down the artery looking for the visual clues one learns to recognize as to the causative problem. I see absolutely nothing. In the meantime, the circulating nurse is starting CPR, awaiting the rest of the cavalry to arrive following a code blue hospital notification. An anaesthetist arrives to perform intubation for ventilatory support. Rounds of drugs are administered as part of CPR protocol, with numerous shocks delivered. Nothing is helping. The room is filling with a dozen nurses and junior doctors. The operating room is notified. A surgeon is called. A short time later I find myself again pushing the bed into an elevator while another cath lab nurse does CPR as we make our way to an operating theatre.

His heart rhythm never recovers. When we arrive there, the surgeon looks at him and merely shakes his head. He knows that there is no coming back from this. He refuses to put the patient on the table. No rhythm. No breathing. No … anything. Mark is gone. One balloon inflation – and everything is changed forever. One 2-mm balloon inflation …

I was certain that I would never be the same again. I never was. But mostly my thoughts were for the members of that family. Their lives would come crashing down. In the midst of emergencies, I have learned to be clear-thinking, decisive, in charge of the room. I do not yell. I remain focused. But that balloon inflation, which would change the course of many lives, nearly ended my career.

Over the years, I have thought about how all doctors, particularly those who perform operative procedures, are affected when those they operate on do not survive. A cardiothoracic or neuro surgeon, an orthopaedist, urologist, general surgeon, gastroenterologist, plastic surgeon – anyone who performs procedures with accompanying risk, including risk of death, is gravely affected by patient mortality during an operation. I want to believe, I do believe, that no honourable or ethical practitioner is not haunted at some level by a mortality, a death in which they played a role. But I will make a distinction here. And I think it is very relevant for those in my line of work. Almost uniformly, those patients under the care of the operators just listed above are under a general anaesthetic when things go terribly wrong. And while I really do not wish to minimize the profound impact of any of these losses, what separates those cases from death on the cath lab table is that our patients are virtually always awake when disaster strikes. To have a patient wheeled into the lab speaking to you, speaking to the staff, to see the unfolding of events leading to loss of consciousness, the loss of blood pressure, the flat line of the ECG, the loss of life in what seems to be in the blink of an eye, is devastating to those involved, from the operator to the nurses to the radiographers. Staff are often left in tears. No one comes to work for this. I would like to say such outcomes are rare. But loss of life in the cath lab is not rare. It is sobering.

After returning back up the elevator, it was, of course, left to me to speak to Mark's wife and son immediately after. They were escorted into a room for privacy. I remained composed and professional. I was honest as to the events as they transpired. I never lie in moments like these. I knew deep in my heart that the decisions were appropriate, even as it was obvious that the outcome was not. I have previously mentioned that I've had to deliver terrible news to those who are effectively strangers to me. It is never easy.

So as they say, this was not my first rodeo. I walked Mark's family through the events as they occurred.

I have watched both the slow and the rapid termination of life. I have seen death more often than I would care to remember. But this was different. I had never been the one that held the instrument, the tool, the weapon, of death. My stories tell of the near misses. The saves. The luck. But until that moment I had never been the causative agent in someone's passing. There would be no good outcome on that day. In today's era, this case would likely have taken five to ten minutes to do, and almost certainly would be successful. It was that simple a case. In the era of balloons, however, nothing was simple.

I sat with Mark's family for some time, knowing that I had forever changed their lives. A woman widowed in her forties, a boy losing his father before puberty was upon him. I held my nerve, my composure, my professionalism. At least what I thought of as professionalism. Once again, I was visited by the guilt. After a period of time, I said my sad goodbyes and directed the family as to the next step, where they could see their husband and father. I walked away from that room to seek solitude. I found an area of the hospital used for those who slept there overnight when on call. I found an empty room, closed the door – and wept. I cried and sobbed for them, for myself, for all things forever changed. My culpability could not be simply set aside knowing that these things happen. I knew all the statistics about risk. It didn't and all these years later, still doesn't matter to me. My role in this death nearly broke me. I don't know how long I stayed in that room and sobbed. I literally don't remember. I only remember thinking that I could not live with this kind of outcome. I could not be culpable ever again. I told myself that if this ever happened again, I was going to quit. I was almost done on that day. I had my own family and their needs to consider. But at that moment, so long ago, nothing else seemed to matter.

As I write this decades later, the guilt still remains. The sadness, the tears can be brought to the surface quite easily. I cannot even begin to count the number of complications and catastrophes that have occurred since. My professional life has been a series of dodging bullets coming my way, and the way of the patient on the table. I have seen many deaths since. But nothing would compare to that day.

What was left for me, after my period of brief mourning, was to change my clothes, and keep moving through the day. The pace of the work constantly leads you to ask, 'What's next?' Years later, I can see that it led me to a life that I would have never imagined.

CHAPTER 8
How did I get into this?

You can't connect the dots looking forward: you can only connect them looking backward. So, you have to trust that the dots will somehow connect in your future.

— Steven Jobs

It's time I take a break from the stories. They can get a bit 'intense', for want of a better term. In fact, in the earlier years of my life, I would never have envisioned, ever, what was to come. I have often been asked if my father or mother was a doctor. Someone else might ask if I had always known that I wanted to do medicine, or when did I decide to choose this profession. But honestly? As I look back, scratching my head, the real question I have asked myself is, how did this ever happen? How did I get here? Because retrospectively, I never saw it coming. Not in a million years.

In the generations preceding mine, there were no professionals within our family. None had attended school beyond year 12. My father and mother were high school graduates, children of immigrants who arrived in the US during the great wave of eastern

European immigration in the early 20th century. They were a product of growing up during the Great Depression in the United States in the late 1920s. Born and raised in the Bronx, they would remain there to raise their own family until retirement.

Following World War II, when my father had fought in France and Germany in the US infantry, he was briefly employed as a dental technician making false teeth. The US economy was rapidly expanding. His cousin was working for a small insurance company in New York and got him a job as a life insurance salesman selling policies door to door in Harlem, where the office was located. For those unfamiliar, Harlem, in those years, was considered a centre of African American music and culture, as well as a black 'ghetto'. It was not uncommon to see famous black musicians or athletes on the streets of Harlem in those years, as I would soon see for myself as a child. On those occasions, when my dad would take me to work with him, I would hang around the office, opening up envelopes, and adding up the monthly insurance premium checks on what would now be thought of as an ancient adding machine. You pushed in the numbered buttons, pulled down the arm on the side of the machine with each entry, and watched the number you put in print on a small roll of paper. Finally, you would ask it for the total sum, magically appearing at the bottom. It would absolutely be considered an antique in today's world.

I was fascinated by that machine. I still marvel at how it added up the numbers. (I'm certain I could figure out the mechanics now, but I prefer to think back and be amazed by the magic.) I was fascinated by everything in the office, from the pointy metal tool I used to open the envelopes, to the swinging wooden door that separated the entrance from where the office workers sat. But mostly I loved watching my father interact with the other salesmen and the office staff. Always constant banter about politics, weather, sports, people. So full of life and humour. Along with his cousin, he would take me out to lunch at the local corner delicatessen, where sour pickles were always on the table, a luxury never otherwise afforded to me. Food was served in 60 seconds and eaten almost that quickly. That's how I remember my visits. Talking, laughing, eating, with every guy in the office trying to be funnier than the next. Talking and jokes was the culture I grew up in.

I also remember those life insurance policies were worth as little as five hundred dollars. Monthly premium checks would arrive worth less than two dollars. Such a small number, even then, but, as Dad explained to me, it was enough for the client to have a casket purchased and get buried, not leaving that burden to their family. His customers were not people of means.

As a teenager, a friend once asked me if my family had money, were we well off. I had never thought about it. I assumed that most people lived in apartments, sharing their bedroom with siblings. Banging on the radiator in the winter for the superintendent to increase the heat. Hanging out the wet laundry on clothes lines straddling the windows across the courtyard in the back of the building. Only then did I come to learn that there were insurance salesmen who made a substantial living. Able to live in the suburbs, buying what we used to call a 'private' house, to be distinguished from a home in an apartment. I can tell you pretty bluntly, affluence was not achieved by selling door to door in Harlem, NY, in the 1950s.

My father had a gift of speaking to people. Obviously, this is a necessary trait as a salesman, particularly when you are knocking on doors. He would banter with waitresses and waiters effortlessly. I once asked him, after we had walked out of a shoe store, how he knew the guy in the shop. He didn't. How did he speak so easily and with such familiarity? He could talk to anyone. I have a photo of him on my bookcase standing next to the then President of the United States, Dwight Eisenhower, in a crowd on the streets of New York. He is literally standing next to the president, wearing a suit and tie! I had to ask, why was he next to the *President of the United States* surrounded by police and workmen? His answer was typical: he was trying to sell him insurance.

He was funny. Well, at least he would remind me how funny he was. But all his friends at the office were funny. It was a great place to hang out as a kid.

My mother was probably ahead of her time. From the time I started primary school she always had a job. She wanted to work. She liked to look nice and dress up during the day. Most of the mothers in our neighbourhood in the Bronx did not have paid employment. It was an era when women, by and large, did not work outside the household. But my mom always worked, and when I was a kid, I had hit the jackpot. My mother worked for the New York Yankees.

The New York Yankees! The powerhouse of professional baseball when I was young. And as a result of Mom's employment there, we had season tickets to the Yankees. When the team started doing promotional events to lure fans to the stadium, like handing out bats and balls, I need not tell you that I was a great beneficiary. I had every autograph of the team and an endless supply of Yankee paraphernalia. My bedroom wall had signed autographed photos by the likes of Mickey Mantle, Whitey Ford, Bobby Richardson, Yogi Berra, Roger Maris … the greats of that era. And not only did I get to see the Yankees when I wanted to, but when the football New York Giants were still playing at Yankee Stadium, my mother was able to get tickets to almost every home season game! This was incredible. Season Giants tickets were so hard to come by that it was said that they were left to people in their wills! Even as a kid with no idea of how the world worked, I knew that in this realm, I really got lucky.

I felt the same way about my neighbourhood. I loved my neighbourhood. This was the baby boom era, and there were a million kids playing in the streets and parks of New York City in the 1950s. We could always get a game of stickball, home run derby, ringolevio, Johnny on the pony (a.k.a buck buck), Russian bulldog, or touch football going. These were the games of our streets. Stoopball (also called off the point), chicken, handball, box baseball, Scully and the games we played that didn't have a name. As an adult, friends would ask if I played tennis or rode horses or surfed as a child. What about fishing or growing vegetables? Skiing? These were things foreign to those of us in the streets of New York. It would be many years into the future before I saw food grow from soil or had the chance to saddle a horse. But a great childhood it was. I would come home from school, throw my stuff into the apartment, and hit the streets. That was where life was for me. It was in the neighbourhood. The absolute last place, the *last place*, I would want to be, was in school. As a kid, I saw school as an interruption of life.

More than just an interruption: I hated school. School was the enemy of a good life. I can honestly look back and see that my primary education was a disaster. It was a combination of being a product of the public New York City school system and my absolute distaste for being there. I virtually never studied. I never read anything beyond comic books. I was not truant – that would have been unacceptable to my parents. Attending school was mandatory, but only a pause in the day before getting back to the neighbourhood.

Yet, somehow, I managed to skip third grade because I reportedly had a high reading level. No idea how that was even possible unless I can attribute it to the power of comic books. Evidence of a brain existed. For me, I just thought one less year of school to worry about. My early education was, for want of a better word, abysmal. And I simply was not interested. It did not get much better.

When I was in the eighth grade, we were required to take a national exam of some kind in the hopes of identifying children who would prosper in higher education, and those who might be better served elsewhere. Following the exams, I was called to see the guidance counsellor at my school. A solidly built man, who was in charge of the wood shop classes, told me quite directly that based on my test score, I would not make it through university. I should consider vocational training. Following high school, I would be better served to develop a trade skill. Imagine that! You are 13 or 14 years old and are being told by your guidance counsellor, an adult with some authority, that you don't appear to be smart enough to get past high school. No parent there. No other adults. Just you and the counsellor. Well, that was that, and to be honest, I could not care less. I wasn't worried about it. I already knew that I didn't trust most adults and I never took anything he said seriously. It wasn't that I was offended or angry or insulted. I just didn't care. School just didn't matter to me, and what my guidance counsellor told me didn't matter either.

By the tenth grade, I was enrolled in what, retrospectively, had to be one of the worst high schools of my era. (I told you things would not get better.) I went to the last public all-boys high school in the city of New York. There were no geographic boundaries for students to attend this school. Students could come from anywhere in the city. This was in the late 1960s, during a time of great racial divisiveness playing out throughout the United States. Martin Luther King was assassinated. Bobby Kennedy was assassinated. John Carlos and Tommie Smith would raise their black-gloved fists on the podium of the Mexico City Olympics in support of Black Power. New York was alive with members flocking to the Black Panthers in support of racial equality. I mention all of this because this was also playing out in my high school. As an all-boys public school with no catchment cut-offs, and a reputation for a strong athletic program, most students who enrolled there were Black and Puerto Rican, coming from all corners of the Bronx and Manhattan, by bus and train. An all-boys school with an estimated enrolment in those days of approximately seven thousand. It was fortunate that the truancy rate was so high! When I graduated three years later, the graduating class was 'only' a thousand. I was a white student in a school dominated by many (not unreasonably) angry young Afro-Americans in the late 1960s. It was not a place of book learning. I learned not to use the bathrooms for fear of being mugged. I learned not to carry any significant sum of money. I learned to watch my back, where to walk, how to walk, where to sit in the cafeteria. Not Shakespeare. Not economics. Not much of anything other than survival, that I can recall.

What can I say at this point? School was not an alluring or attractive place, and I was the recipient of neither guidance nor inspiration to learn. Within a couple of years of leaving high school, I could not remember the name of even one teacher I had interacted with. I never even knew the name of the principal of the school. I have so many friends and family members who, decades later, remember teachers, aides, principals of schools they attended. They reminisce about their school friends, school functions, activities that they shared during their high school years. I remember nothing. I remember no one. And nothing about learning. I remember being jumped by three guys looking for money on my first day of high school. I remember a guy with a hook for a hand (yes, a hook, like Captain Hook in Peter Pan) waving it in my face while being surrounded by four others. I remember ransoming a friend, who was grabbed by five others while walking home, for two dollars. What I remember I have put to paper here. This was my time in high school. It merely reinforced what I had been carrying with me since I first walked into primary education: school was an interruption of life. I hated school.

What would follow next was university. Despite my parents having no education beyond high school, it seemed that in our generation, it was almost expected you would continue with school as the path to a better life than they had. I didn't give it much thought. My older sister went to college (what Australians would call university) in the city while living at home, and so I figured I would also go, as a matter of course. Unlike her, however, I definitely wanted to live away from home. There was nothing left for me in the Bronx. The neighbourhood had changed, people had moved away, and the games of my childhood had given way to new things.

I was fortunate to get into a school within the state university system, making the costs far more affordable than a private school. I secretly would have loved to have gone to an Ivy League school. I had once visited Yale where the New York Giants were having a practice session, and I could not get over how great the campus looked! (It was never about the education.)

I was fortunate in some ways. In my less-than-higher-learning high school, I was ranked as a good student getting relatively good grades despite my overall indifference and absence of study. This is what got me into a state university: being near the top of a class of the barely literate! But then it happened. I failed my first university exam. Abysmal failure at that. I had never failed an exam before, despite never studying. I was stunned. I was not only stunned, but I was also scared. Because I had no idea, no clue how to fix this. Using the minimal 'tools' of learning at my disposal, it was obvious that at this level I could not succeed. I may not have cared about being educated, but I certainly did care about succeeding in whatever I was involved with. But I had no other tools available to do better than this failure! Yet this moment would lead me to a new chapter. I would learn the first great lesson that would help me through all that would follow.

It was a friend who would change it all for me. I gradually would learn a method of grasping and understanding the subject matter. And yes, there was a method to this. Prior to that, it was all about what I could memorize, or what seemed instinctually obvious to me. But in that first year of university life, having failed my first exam, ever, I would learn how to learn.

My great friend Bruce, who would forever remain my best friend from that first year in university, was a slower student than I (I am hopeful, and pretty certain that he would agree to this without any insult intended.) But it was his method of study, and our developing friendship, that would define the way I began to discern and understand the written word. A way that I would continue to use for the rest of my life. We sat together, lived together, studied together, and taught one another the material that needed to be learned. We examined, explained, verbalized until we understood the material at hand. It became clear to me from those early years that until you can teach something to another, you are not truly versed. I believe, no, I *know*, that the reason why we both became the teachers we would later become was those early years of study. I happened to be at the right place at the right time. It took that friendship from over fifty years ago to get me started on a path. One friendship made all the difference.

Or let's just say that ultimately, yeah, it would make a difference. But not quite yet. While I was busy learning to learn, and becoming more successful as a student, my interests were still not in the world of education or that of any professional degree. I wanted to be a gym teacher. I wanted to 'play' for the rest of my life. I became an oarsman while attending university, an endeavour I would continue for over a decade. It was a central part of my life. I would have been content to spend my hours training at the gym and to spend my life teaching sports.

It's funny how the small, little things in life add up and change the course of what is to be. I was not close to my sister in those days. She was four years older and had a very different kind of relationship with our parents than I did. We shared a bedroom until she was 17 years old, not an age for a teenage girl to welcome sharing a room with a younger brother. We had grown apart years earlier and only spoke to each other on occasion if I called home and she was there. Somehow, during this period of time when I began to contemplate my future, we had a conversation on the phone. The memory is vivid. I doubt she would even remember what to her was perhaps a trivial comment. When I told her I was thinking of becoming a physical education teacher, she told me that I would be wasting my life. She thought that I was too smart for such a career choice, and I could do more with my life (I would hope no gym teachers are insulted at this moment).

My sister had never said anything positive to me in our entire existence. *Never.* She was telling me that I was smart. Whaaaat?

Maybe, I thought, just maybe, she was on to something. Maybe I should think this through. It is crazy to look back and realize that I really never equated how 'smart' one was with what to do with one's life. How simplistic and naïve. But because of that conversation and a thought that she implanted, I decided to hold off on pursuing a degree in physical education. It was another singular moment that would change the course of this life.

I had now graduated with a four-year degree in biology. It was a fairly useless degree to say the least. I had managed to achieve a very high grade point average despite my early failure, having been nearly a straight-A student in the sciences for four years. I had been a varsity athlete throughout, rowing with the university crew team. I had graduated magna cum laude and received entrance into Phi Beta Kappa, an honour society demarcated by one's academic achievements. In a university of over twenty thousand students, I had been awarded a student athlete scholarship by the Dean of the University for my achievements, and my photo was in the newspaper alongside the dean and the family sponsoring the scholarship. My father was proud. My mother was proud. I had set the scene.

I thought of myself as a relatively uneducated man. I had not read books. I knew nothing of the world, politics, history, art … Other than being a good student with exemplary grades and a fierce desire to train and compete, I was not really accomplished at anything. I would turn 22 years of age before I picked up a book and read it cover to cover. I had never read a complete book while in school. Looking back nearly five decades later, I could almost weep for that young man and how little he knew.

It was only much later that I came to realize how important teachers and mentors are to the young. How one person can make all the difference in the direction or path one takes, even the dreams that one has. I loved my mother and father. And I know they loved me too. As a child and a young man, my father was the only man I truly respected and would listen to. Yet, I had no mentors during my years of education.

Following my university graduation, there were no more student loans to help me pay the bills. I was out of school, with no idea what would happen next. It was then I was essentially forced to move back home to the Bronx and live with my parents. Having lived away for the past four years, moving back with my mother and father felt like I had become a miserable, abject failure. My friends were all gone. I had no plans for the future. I applied for a job as an orderly at the closest hospital, but even in this I was turned down. Despite whatever trivial success I had as a student, there was nothing on the horizon. It was during this return home, with no vision of what was to come next, that my father, somewhat pained and nearly in tears, told me that he had failed me. In his desire to provide the guidance and direction for a life he saw his son wasting, he was both confused and wounded. This man, who I loved more than anyone in the world, was upset in a way that I had never seen in him. At the time, I could not relate to nor understand his grief. I was not worried about myself and did not 'get' why he was. It would not be until many years later, as a father, that I could comprehend the sorrow and the helplessness he must have felt at that moment to say such a thing. For I had never thought he had failed me. He had given me his gift of speaking to others, and of humour. I would later put both to good use.

Having spent the summer months living back in the Bronx, it

was obvious that this could not continue. No friends. No job. No prospects. It was then that I elected to return to my university town and find work. And now, after all of this, I was to find myself working in a construction job pouring concrete. Out of school, working a seasonal temporary job with absolutely no idea what I was going to do with my life. Other temporary jobs would ensue once the weather was too cold (this being the northeast US) to work outdoors in the building trade. One such part-time job was delivering newspapers door to door. I would go to the office where the newspapers were distributed and see adult couples filling up pickup trucks with newspapers. It hadn't dawned on me that for some, this was serious money that 'grown-ups' needed to live on day to day.

I, on the other hand, was sharing a place with three other guys, living the life of what I have often called 'a bum'. One day as I was walking through a neighbourhood, hanging papers on doorknobs, I found myself being chased by a dog – the classic delivery outcome going from door to door in a leafy neighbourhood in upstate New York. It was in this singular moment that again, my life would change forever. As I was running down the street with a sack of newspapers around my shoulder, contemplating the absurdity of the scene unfolding, I had the realization that nobody, anywhere, cared about anything I thought I had accomplished. No one was interested that I was a stellar student. Nobody was intrigued that I was a competitive athlete with trophies and medals, or cared if I delivered newspapers for the rest of my life! Anything that I had accomplished in my life was of absolutely no meaning or importance to anyone in that neighbourhood, or anywhere else for that matter. A light bulb lit up in my head: it all seemed intuitively obvious to me now. I had been living a life of make-believe, waiting for the universe to bestow its wisdom, its decision on how my life was to play out. I immediately saw that the only way out for me was through education. For a guy who never really cared about school or the educational process, this was to be a defining moment. I didn't know what to do next, or even how to go about becoming educated. But I knew it was time for me to go back to school and figure it out.

Within a couple of months, I managed to become a non-matriculating student. I started taking science courses at the graduate-school level without receiving any credit towards a degree. When I began taking courses, I applied to a master's program in immunology, working at the prestigious local cancer centre. I was accepted after a semester and continued with my studies. While taking a course in physiology, I discovered that there were students in the class who were being fully funded. Again, whaaat? They were on a full-fee scholarship with a living stipend to go with it in one of the doctoral programs in the university. This was almost too good to be true. I was fortunate that with my previous studies at this university, along with my scholarship award to graduate school, I was accepted into the PhD program in the Department of Pathology, studying the nature of muscular dystrophy. And so, for the next four years, I would be paid to study while I would forge a potential career path. At least in theory …

It was not smooth going for me. Why should this come as a surprise? While I sought out an education, I remained resistant to those who sought to educate me. I simply could not 'connect' at any level with my professors. My advisor during my time in the master's program told me that I would never amount to anything. (Sigh.) It was his opinion that I did not have the work ethic to be successful. I understand why he thought that. I just didn't enjoy the work. Having left the master's program in immunology, now two to three years later and halfway through my PhD program, another stumble. I was put on suspension. It was not for my studies. More for my attitude. I spent a lot of time pursuing more enjoyable aspects of life when I should have been in the pathology lab. I was deeply involved with my physical training as my rowing life took centre stage. My suspension in the PhD program required extra research time, in a second lab, spent far from school campus, but I was not about to give up yet. Despite two simultaneous projects being required of me at the time, I struggled and limped through my doctorate.

When asked what my PhD is in, my reply has always been consistent. It is in Perseverance. I wanted to quit so often. Years of research in a pathology lab, utilizing tools such as scanning and electron microscopy, and immunoelectrophoresis, alongside the unpleasantness of animal sacrifice for tissue analysis. Followed, ultimately, by a formal written thesis and oral defence of that thesis. Writing a doctoral thesis is hard. It was very hard for me. Long days in the library, months at a time, many years before the internet. Isolation and loneliness. My father warned me that quitting was often a formula for more quitting in the future. That was not me. I pushed on. And finally, after a total of five years of graduate school, I managed to write and orally defend my PhD in front of our departmental committee. I was terribly relieved. I was exhausted by it all.

I had learned many things in the pursuit of my PhD. I learned to read research articles. I learned many technical skills. Most importantly, I acquired a critically thinking mind, able to analyse and question research conclusions. This skillset would serve me well in the years to come. Unfortunately, one of the things I also ended up learning was that being a basic science researcher was not for me. This career path was to end. I had to find another. Five years it took, to learn what I did not want.

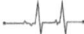

During that final year of graduate studies, I began to apply to medical schools. Many of the classes that were required in my PhD pursuits overlapped with the medical school curriculum. And I believed I had a gift for communication, the gift from my father. With that ability, I thought that a career requiring good communication skills, rather than laboratory research, might suit me better. In my naïve state of mind, I wanted to 'make a difference' in the world, the specifics of that thought being completely ambiguous. I not only had my university awards and honour societies, but also a PhD. I believed I was an ideal candidate for acceptance.

I applied to sixty-one medical schools, and I was accepted into … one. Even the university where I had done all my studies, where I had earned my doctorate, rejected me. (To this day I have no confirmation, but I suspect I was blackballed by one of my professors who truly disliked me.) But nevertheless, one school took me. Quite remarkable yet again how just one thing changes a life. One great friend, one light-bulb moment, one sibling conversation, one acceptance. So many speed bumps along the way.

One of my fondest memories is calling my mother and father, who had by then retired and gone to live in Florida, as so many retirees from the northeast US did in that era. I used to call on Sundays, collect. My mother would become seriously angry with me if I failed to call: there was no way to know if your child was okay without a phone call! The morning that I received that acceptance letter into medical school, I decided to call my parents. During the week, no less! My mother answered the phone and immediately became very concerned when she heard my voice. 'What's the matter?' were her first words. I couldn't help myself. I had to feed into the worry, draw out the suspense. I timidly asked her if I could borrow $40,000 (an approximate tuition cost, equivalent to $160,000 today). Her voice dropped softer as she asked me, 'What happened?'

'Well,' I said, 'I just … got into MEDICAL SCHOOL!'

After uttering those words, what I remember hearing next was hyperventilation into the phone. And her yelling for my father. Her joy was palpable. For my parents, products of the Great Depression, lower-middle-class working people, having me become a medical doctor was a hope of a lifetime. This is a sentiment I am certain exists around the world for working-class parents who pray for their children's success. They cried into the phone their happiness for me and for themselves. My father could now know he had not failed his son. He could spend the next years casually dropping the 'my son the doctor' line on those he targeted. My mother went one better by buying a T-shirt that said *My son the doctor, doctor* (MD, PhD). It seemed to be the culmination of long years of searching and frustration.

Yes, I went to medical school. I would graduate with many academic honours. I would go on to do my medical residency and ultimately my fellowship in cardiology. From college graduation until the finish of my fellowship would take me *sixteen* years. During those years I would have twin sons. I would become more educated. I would read books. I would retire from rowing. It was time to put playing aside and join the working world with all the hours that medical training would require. I would need to moonlight nights and weekends when not on call to support the family – many hours working in emergency rooms or ICUs to supplement my income. For five years of residency and fellowship I needed a second job, only adding to the burden of taking on-call shifts.

Over the years I have been fascinated by, and at times envied, those who from an early age seem to know their path in life. Some are destined for athletic brilliance, encouraged and nurtured at a young age. There are those whose families have set them on to a successful business venture. Others that took to technology early in life and became successful in the new industries developed since the birth of the internet. I was not one of those. I never knew what I was to do with my time here.

One friend. One dog. One school. One sister. Life sometimes seems a series of one-moments, singular dots, linked together to ultimately form a chain of events. A chain, once created, that points to the pathway forward. I felt as if I had gotten over the hump of life. Many challenges in the past, and a bright future ahead.

And yet, the long years of searching and frustration were not done. I thought that getting into medicine was the end of my search. I didn't know it would just lead to another road where the path to discovery would begin anew. But that is another part of this story.

CHAPTER 9
The break

Rock bottom became the solid foundation on which I rebuilt my life.

— J.K. Rowling

At this stage of my story, I must jump forward in time. I had now been in practice nearly fifteen years. There had been wins and there had been losses, successes and disappointments. I had my share of excitement and, unfortunately, far too much monotony. I was no longer happy with the day-to-day of life. Truth be told, I was a bit of a mess.

My personal life had become unstable, and my professional life, tiresome. 'Making the donuts' seemed to have become more the norm. The excitement was ebbing and what I was doing day to day was no longer rewarding or enjoyable. I suspect that any number of people who have been employed in the same job for a similar number of years begin to fatigue of the daily workload set upon them. For those fortunate enough to either love what they do forever, or change employment to something fresh and different, perhaps this timeline is not relevant. But like many others, I had reached a point where something needed to change. I must add that I was not alone in this. The number of physicians that I knew in the community who were tired by the 'work', looking forward to a time when they no longer had to, was far more than you might imagine. I heard all the complaints. I also knew that most would never really do anything about it. After all, people like to complain, particularly when there is a sense of a shared grievance.

I hoped I had brought good things to the patients. I wasn't even certain of that. I was bored and tired and becoming increasingly depressed that after all of the years it took to get this far, I was not enjoying it any longer. I had become professionally stagnant and was no longer learning anything new despite all the advancements taking place. The exciting moments were too infrequent to keep my attention. I believed the problem was not merely too many years in the same job; it was the nature of the practice that I'd found myself joining those many years earlier, when my priority was settling down in one place and beginning to start a stable life with a comfortable income. But now it felt that I had reached a place of professional mediocrity, with no hope of ever being more than I was. Was this it, for the rest of my life?

I had chosen a path to financially support my family, and unfortunately, for me, this came at a cost of arrested professional development. I had stopped reading. I had stopped attending professional meetings. I was there to work and make a living. Deep in my private thoughts was a lingering disappointment with myself. When did mediocrity become ... me?

This all became crystal clear to me when one day I was in the office seeing a man I had known for many years. I had performed multiple coronary interventions on him, spread over several years. He was finally feeling well and healthy. I clearly remember coming out of the exam room when he turned to me to shake my hand yet again and thank me for all I had done to preserve his health and his life. He was a very decent guy, and I actually truly liked him. I can still see his face. But it was what came next that had an everlasting, and somewhat damaging effect on me. A person, a man I liked, sharing these kind and appreciative thoughts. Thoughts that should be received with equal gratitude for the privilege of his trust. It's part of the pleasure of the job: feeling as if you've done something worthwhile and tangibly relevant for another. Moments like these are a large part of why we do what we do and help us feel a part of the wider human community. Yet, despite his thanks and appreciation, I felt … nothing. The worst thing that I could have at that moment: *absolutely no reaction* to what he had said. A man thanks you for a gift that has such significance to him, and you feel nothing. It was worse than that – it just did not matter to me. It wasn't that I wished him ill; it simply didn't matter. Another day, another donut made. I was losing my connection to others.

Please don't misinterpret my reaction. At some level I *was* pleased that he was feeling well. I really was. As I said, I liked this man, and his medical problems were under good control following successful coronary interventions over years of time. But within my own emotional framework, whatever that was, it seemed to matter very little. It was probably more important to me that I hadn't done anything bad to him. No lawsuits to contend with. No hassles to shrug off. I knew at that moment, so many years ago, that I was broken inside. My emotional connection to the work, to the people, to the staff was broken. *I* was very, very broken. What I didn't realize at the time that this was all part of a pattern of social isolation (common among men, but that is another topic) that had begun years earlier and that now had spread to all corners of my life. To very bad effect.

I have learned over the years not to internalize the thanks I receive, never allowing them to have me believe that I am 'better' than I am. It is so easy to fall into that ego trap, as I have clearly seen happen to many others over time. The thanks are the reward. But to feel nothing? To suddenly confront the fact that I was no longer emotionally connected to my work, the patient, or the outcomes? It was a breaking point for me. I was not the same after that day. I continued to work for a time, but I knew that the end was coming near. I was going through the motions. Life had gotten the better of me, and I was sinking.

The details of my leaving the practice are not relevant here, but it was quite obvious that my focus had drifted and it was time to find a new life. I was exhausted and numbed by being on call 180 days per year, every year, which by now had extended to well over a decade. I was irritated by practicing in a litigious environment when it seemed everyone was watching over my shoulder. The patients, the families, the hospital utilization services, administration, nurses, colleagues (better said, competitors). I walked about as if there was a professional bullseye on my back just waiting for someone to hit the centre with a poison arrow.

I did not want to be a doctor any longer. Whatever my weaknesses and strengths have been, following along on a path that was not of my own choosing was not for me. Practicing medicine in the United States was becoming less appealing as health care was becoming more and more monetized (it always had been, but it was getting incrementally worse), and independent small groups like mine were becoming a thing of the past. My family had fractured, and I had to force myself each day to do the work.

I knew that I was done, and I saw no option but to close this chapter of my life and hope, just hope, that another chapter would begin. It has been said that until you close the door behind you, you cannot see the others that are available for you to open. It was not an easy decision to leave after all the years of education and training that led me here. Leaving, after all that it had taken for me to find both a career and a safe and secure place to live. And yet that's exactly what I did. I resigned. I left my profession, with very little to show for it.

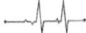

I was separated, had been for nearly a decade, living alone. There were no longer any serious relationships to consider. Whatever relationships I tried to bring to life during that decade had ended as my spiral into isolation became worse and worse. By this time, my sons were living away from home studying at universities. I made certain first that the education of my boys was financially taken care of, leaving me with little else.

I spent time riding horses, white-water kayaking, backpacking in the mountains, ice skating: so many pursuits unknown to me as a child. I even spent time in an organization that has since been labelled as a cult (I was wise enough to exit before law enforcement descended). I pondered a future with no clue what would happen next.

I thought of becoming a white-water rafting guide, an expert witness for medical liability cases, becoming a coroner. I thought of moving to the mountains, to a log cabin. Maybe a beach in the Caribbean pouring drinks at a straw-thatched roof bar (not serious). I had no idea what was next. Other than medicine, I had no skills and no knowledge. Too old to start a mountain guiding company, no idea on how to become a coroner. Major dislike of medical lawsuits and those who practice them daily. What was next? It is difficult for me to express in writing how lost and how alone I felt at this time of my life, even when there were those who held out their hands to help.

Six months passed by, and I happened to see a small advertisement in a medical journal – it could not have been longer than four lines. What I was doing even looking in a medical journal remains a mystery to me. What I had seen was an advertisement from a company that temporarily placed American doctors in positions all over the world, with a specialty for placements in Australia. Australia? I had never thought about Australia – as a place to be, let alone a place to live. But I must confess that it caught my eye.

Another one of those singular moments was about to occur. I had just finished a book by Bill Bryson titled *Down Under*. Mr Bryson has written many stories of his travels in various parts of the world. For those who have not read his books, his style is soft comedy, laced with fascinating anecdotes of places and people. My recollection of the first chapter, when he initially arrives for his visit to Australia, was his reflections on all the various ways there were for nature to kill you, be it on land or in the water. It is a country of, let us say, *unusual* animals and insects. Because of its physical isolation on the world map, the flora and fauna can be quite unique, leading the country to have developed some of the most stringent biohazard laws in the world. For instance, it is home to two of only five species of egg-laying mammals in the world: the platypus, and the short-beaked echidna. (The three other species of long-beaked echidna are all endemic to Papua New Guinea.)

Strangely enough, Bryson's description of Australia and his travels there fascinated me. Notably the comical take on what can end your life. And so, when I saw this advertisement from a locum company, I thought, why not give it a shot? I didn't think they would have anything for me anyway. My skill set is quite specific, and I was not interested in doing general cardiology or general medicine. But I elected to send them an email regardless, during a time when email was still in its infancy (or at least for me).

My life continued somewhat aimlessly. I was still paddling the rivers, hiking the trails, and riding horses twice weekly. And while these activities provided me with some forms of entertainment they were, by and large, done alone. Once I had resigned, my life was lived very much alone. Despite the relationships I had formed with others over the years, much like with the patients, I simply could not connect normally. It was not a happy time.

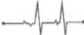

Approximately two months later I received a return email from the locum company, offering a position for one year in Australia. *One year?* No way was I going to leave the safety of my home, as depressing as it felt, to go around the globe for a whole year. I had never travelled that far. For that matter, I had never travelled outside the US. I had no idea what the job entailed. I was not even interested in being a doctor. I only thought this was a way to parlay my degree to do something else. When I inquired where the job would be, I was told it was in Tasmania. What? Where? I thought they were talking about employment in Australia! Where the hell is Tasmania? I had to look it up on a map (pre–Google Maps) and was at least assured that it was part of Australia, even if it was a few hundred kilometres south of the mainland, separated by water. I had this vision of a backward island with minimal electricity and buildings with no windows (it is truly embarrassing, if not amusing, to admit to all this years later). I baulked. I tried to search for some information about Tasmania, but the internet was not what it is today, and there was not a lot of information to feed upon.

I went ahead and accepted the interview, at least curious to find out what this was all about. I was interviewed for the job via a long-distance phone call in the early morning hours, given the sixteen-hour time difference. Following a brief chat, I was invited to come to work. Despite my own unease, I continued the process of applying. There was lots of paperwork to be completed, something I would never have accomplished without the help of the locum company. Part of the requirements was to prove that I could speak English! I said on the phone, 'You are talking to me, is that not enough proof?'

'No.' A simple answer. I had to submit proof that I had been educated in English by providing a high school diploma, something I had not seen in decades. I ultimately had to contact my high school in the Bronx and ask them if they had records from over thirty years ago, proving I had graduated from there. I was stunned that such a record was provided! Despite my high school education being somewhat limited, at least in the end they came through for me.

So, after all the paperwork was done, which was a process that stretched over months, I was scheduled to fly to Tasmania and begin my employment. I was full of hesitation and concern, but I had negotiated a contract that would last only three months. I could not fathom going around the world to a place that I didn't know, had never seen, and living there longer than that. The reservations were made, and I was due to fly out weeks before Christmas.

I emphasize that at this point, I was a bit …worried. Was I out of my mind? I had never met anyone who had left the US to live elsewhere. I know that this is now commonplace around the globe, but it was not common where I came from. If my mother and father had still been alive, I feel certain that they would have thought I needed serious professional help (and by that, I mean, psychiatric).

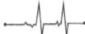

The day comes to leave, and the weather is bad. Really bad. Trees are blowing sideways and it's pouring rain. Not having been a good traveller on a good day, I panic and cancel everything. I'm not going. The entire expedition was a foolish and immature idea, and I should seriously be rethinking my decision. I call the locum company and tell them that the weather is atrocious, I cannot get on the plane. Despite some level of embarrassment in making this call, part of me begins to think that this may be *the* great excuse to exit from this whole ridiculous, ludicrous plan!

Unfortunately for me, I am surprised to find the woman on the other end of the phone so understanding. Maybe there were other lunatics like me afraid of flying in bad weather and more afraid of going to Australia. She calmly tells me that it's quite alright, and when do I want to leave? For a second time, I am thinking, this is my chance! With a few well-spoken and apologetic words, I can bail out of this crazy idea of flying to the other side of the world where I know no one. On the other hand, I'm also thinking that this woman is going to think I am a coward. Given the time and effort it has taken to get all the necessary paperwork done to get me this gig, bailing out because of bad weather really has the look of true cowardice. I don't want to be thought a coward. I don't like the look. So, I bravely rebook to go a few days later and hang up the phone, somewhat crestfallen. I had my out. I cracked and gave in. I am now 'forced' to follow through with the plan. I know, I forced myself. It was easier to blame the kind woman on the phone. If only she hadn't been so nice …

And so, days later, with the weather having subsided, I boarded the first of what would be four flights taking a total of thirty-six hours to reach my ultimate destination in Launceston, Tasmania. Thirty-six hours! The longest flight I had ever previously been on was five hours. I had not slept. I arrived to a hot, dry climate in December, having left the coolness of the northeast US at that time of year.

While flying over Tasmania, I had my eyes peeled, looking out the window searching for signs of civilization. I kid you not when I say that I saw absolutely no sign of any life. There was a lot of greenery, trees, grass, et cetera. No houses. Rolling hills looking like a good place for a Hobbit community to live. But no signs of human activity. Retrospectively, I was likely just sitting on the wrong side of the plane, but as it circled and came about for its landing, I had yet to see a house or anything resembling a community of any kind. My worries were deepening.

The airport is one where there is no walkway pushed to the plane. You descend the steps onto the tarmac. There were friends and family members awaiting their visitors, standing on the tarmac, waving, separated from those arriving by little more than a rail. There was none of the security that the US instituted following the incidents of 9/11. That was to come later. I walked to the carousel to get my baggage. There was no carousel. A little trolley car pulled up with all the bags in tow and a sniffer dog jumped up on the bags and began his rounds of … sniffing. That done, everyone just went out and grabbed their bag off the trolley.

I should note, by the way, that the sniffer dogs in Tasmania are not sniffing for weapons or explosives; they are there for biosecurity. They specialize in finding fresh fruit or nuts in your baggage. Australia is very strict about foreign organisms being brought into the country, and Tasmania is strict about mainland products being brought to the island state. To this day, you might have a Glock pistol under your jacket and get past the dogs, but be ready to be brought down if you have fresh oranges or cashews in your pocket (only kidding – sort of).

I was met at the airport by one of the secretaries from the Department of Medicine at the hospital employing me. After collecting my baggage, my first error was, of course, getting into the car on the wrong side. My driver turned to me and said, 'Probably best if I do the driving at this stage, Brian.' This would occur many times over the months ahead. After switching seats, I was driven out of the airport heading to town, a town I had yet to lay my eyes upon, even when I was thousands of feet above it.

I was still quite concerned as we left the airport, continuing to see nothing. Oh yes, there was a llama farm across the street from the airport. Or maybe it was sheep. Somehow, that did not bring great comfort or joy at that moment. The area around the airport in Launceston has been significantly developed over the ensuing years, but when I first arrived, there was simply nothing there. We entered onto a highway, yet still, nothing. I had already begun to formulate an escape plan of how to leave and go home. If not for the fact I was seriously jetlagged, miserable, and disoriented after this trying flight, I do believe I would have looked for the next flight out. However, about fifteen minutes from leaving the airport, I was relieved to see the makings of a moderate-sized town, with lots of buildings and many more people. We drove past a McDonalds as we entered, a sure sign of civilization in the 21st century. I don't recall speaking much in the car, likely being in a state of some shock and not having slept in over thirty-six hours.

Our first stop was the hospital where I would be working in the months ahead. Public hospital systems were a bit new to me, coming from the US where the only comparable hospital system is that created by the Veterans' Administration. This health care system is provided for those veterans who choose to continue hospital and outpatient medical care there. I had spent some of my fellowship training in one of the VA hospitals in the northeast, and I must say it was not where I would have chosen to receive health care. But in Australia, the public system is another thing, and I had been hired to work in the public hospital here in Launceston for a minimal and laughable salary. But this was about the adventure (or so I told myself).

I remember quite vividly my first impressions of the hospital. Let us say my misgivings about my decision to come were not alleviated. It appeared to me as an old building, more like a concrete block that could house felons than a modern hospital. I was not trying to be judgemental, but first impressions are what they are, and this one stayed with me. The building was, in fact, not that old, having been rebuilt twenty years earlier, but with governmental austerity in mind, to serve as a general hospital for the community.

I was willing to accept what was on offer.

What followed contributed further to the feeling of insanity that my decision to take this position seemed to suggest. I was driven to the apartment being provided for me by the hospital as part of the contract for the next three months. Along with the apartment came an automobile, one in which I would have further adventures as I learned to negotiate driving on the other side of the road.

The apartment was in a good location in town, no more than minutes away from the hospital, with a nice view out the back. As to the apartment itself, however, I was stunned at what I suppose I would have called its threadbare condition. Minimal furniture, minimal heating for the months ahead if needed, no air conditioner for the summer (granted, I was to learn that is not particularly necessary in Tasmania), and worn, outdated kitchen appliances. It was small, and I would say I would not have paid more than two hundred dollars for everything in the apartment: all the furniture, all the bedding, all the utensils. It was very, very basic, providing the same vibes I had when living as a student many years ago. But, again, while I continued to question my sanity, I did not wish to be judgemental. Perhaps, I thought, this was how the average person lived in Tasmania. Perhaps this was the norm. (Spoiler alert: not true. I was living in a dump.)

The secretary left me to settle in, and I was alone. Alone on the other side of the planet, at the bottom of the earth, at the end of the line. Nothing much further south other than birds and Antarctica. I was a long way from home, and I didn't know a soul. Social media had yet to be invented. I didn't know what time it was across the globe or even how to make a phone call to a friend or to my sons in the US. I sat in that tiny living room on a solitary piece of furniture, staring at my suitcase, and thought, *what have I done?*

CHAPTER 10
The start of something new

The first step towards getting somewhere is to decide you're not going to stay where you are.

— J.P. Morgan

Leaving one's country of birth is not an easy decision for anyone. It was particularly unnerving for me given I was already more than halfway through life. All my family and friends were in the United States. My sons were there.

Moving was a challenging time, both emotionally and physically. Deconstructing a life with all its webs of complexity and starting anew was the task I was faced with. What yet remained for me in the midst of making this decision was speaking with my sons. They were then halfway through their university studies. Moving so great a distance from them was, and remains, the most difficult decision I have ever made. It wasn't just the decision that was made more than twenty years ago. It has been living with it. In the great emotional turmoils of my life, they were the two things, the two people, that kept me sane and grounded. They were a constant. More than once, I have wondered how I would have survived if not for them. The responsibilities of work and children can be a weight so heavy, days that seem insurmountable, that there were moments that I wished for an easier, earlier time of life. Yeah, responsibilities of adulthood and parenthood can be so, so tough. Exhausting. Demanding. And yes, relentless. Bills to pay, timelines to be met, commitments to others whether at home or at work. The responsibilities of having my sons, however, likely saved my life. Making dinners, school lunches, picking up or dropping off, wrestling on the floor, watching stupid shows on TV, laughing, and I mean serious laughing watching the Simpsons ... No matter what, in this I would not break. The link from my father, through me to them, could not, must not be broken.

Some parents, perhaps, might wonder what emotional scars they inevitably leave their children, no matter how they are raised or what challenges they face. Having moved across the globe, far from their daily lives, has made me keenly aware of the scars that I may have created. And so it was, so many years ago now, that I sat with the both of them on a beach outside of Boston and told them all that had to be said. I have never known, as I write this, whether my sons knew of or could have understood the unhappiness, the stagnation that I had felt for many years. It was something I think most parents try to shield their children from. The difficulties of adulthood need not be shared with those too young to process this kind of information. Yet not for a moment were they anything but supportive of my choice, despite the closeness that binds us. And the distance that would separate us. I could have made different decisions earlier in life, better decisions. In so many ways I was not prepared to take on the responsibilities of adulthood. Yet with my sons, it was a debt to my father, long gone, that had to be repaid. I hope I got it right.

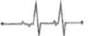

How does one start again when already mid-way through life? Let alone far from home, no family about, no friends known, minimal financial resources, on the other side of the planet. This undoubtedly was on my mind as I wandered the streets of Launceston during those early days following my arrival.

Millions of people migrate around the world seeking a better life, be it for family, work, education, safety, or economics. It is common. Yet, I would never have envisioned that one day this would be me. Despite the US being the proverbial 'melting pot' of the world, when I lived there, much of the ethnic and cultural mix seemed diluted by the sheer size of the population, along with socioeconomic differences, and the often-seen clustering of immigrants within their 'own' communities. There, it was as if this immigrant part of the work force just 'blended' in. I simply never noticed. Joining the workforce in a hospital in Launceston, Tasmania was different. It seemed almost akin to working at the United Nations. There were staff members from all over the globe. From countries I knew little of. They were not an 'invisible' part of the community. I was to find myself working with, and teaching, junior doctors from all over the world.

Prior to my arrival, I had never worked closely with anyone who I knew had moved to or from another country. Or maybe I simply hadn't noticed. During my New York upbringing, I was surrounded by second generation ethnic groups and many African Americans, but I didn't know anyone who had immigrated to the US and 'started again'. And more strikingly, I had not known of a single person who had left the US to live in another country. The term 'expatriate' was a word known to me, but in word only.

Why would someone leave the United States and live in another country? Why would one choose to leave the land of freedom and opportunity? Why? These were my thoughts many years ago. Seems crazy to think that now. But then, that was the way my mind worked. For me, this was all new. And a bit unsettling.

I was fortunate enough to have a profession, and a specialized skill set, that had taken many years to acquire. I was even luckier that there was somewhere in the world that sought that skill set and knowledge. It was not lost upon me, however, that I had no desire to work in that job or apply that skill set. I had decided to leave it behind me when I left my employment, now over eight months before. And yet here I was, hired to do just that, to get 'back on the horse' and do the work again. Far from home, far from my sons, I felt, again, alone.

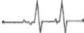

Well, it helped to know the language. At least everyone spoke English. That was a major obstacle overcome. Of course, the trunk of the car is the boot; the hood is the bonnet; buying something that is dear is not an endearment (it's expensive); you do *not* root for your friend's daughter in the spirit of sportsmanship. Arvo is afternoon; a barbie is what you throw the shrimp on along with hamburgers, steaks, et cetera; bathers are swimming suits; brekky is breakfast; buggered is really tired; and you do not call it a fanny pack, but a bum bag (both rooting and fanny are specific coarse references to sexual matters). A slab is a cartoon of beer, and a sheila is a woman. Australians like to end as many words as possible with a 'y' sound, so mosquito is mozzie, sweets are lollies, footy is football, a sickie is a day off for being sick – it's a long list. And when you get the lingo down, then 'Bob's your uncle'! (i.e., everything is fine). I used to keep a list of all the words but eventually abandoned the project, knowing that in time it would all make sense. Besides, these were not serious issues to overcome like learning a language from the beginning.

Of course, there was the day when how to pronounce the word did become an issue.

One of my first working days at the hospital, a woman was bleeding out of her right arm from a site that had been punctured by a cannula. There was nothing to panic about. I just told the nurse to put on a tourniquet. She stared at me. I repeated, 'Put on a tourniquet'. She stared, looking for support around the room. I said, 'Don't you guys know what a tourniquet is?' I was somewhat surprised, after all, this was a first world nation. At least I thought it was. Now, I am saying, 'The thing you wrap on an arm tightly?' After a moment, they responded (excuse my misspelling), '*Oh*, a tor-ni-kay!' and proceeded to apply one to the patient's arm.

My 'tur-na-kit', as pronounced in the US, is their 'tor-ni-kay' (as if the French had colonized the island instead of the English!) So, the language lessons were coming along quite nicely.

Moving to another country that is a member of the British Commonwealth can also entail taking measures to avoid being hit by a passing automobile.

I was walking down the street on one of my first days in town and was about to cross this fairly narrow street. As I stepped off the kerb, I felt an arm grab me and pull me back while a car whisked by … coming from my right. Ah, yes, driving on the other side of the road! When crossing, or driving and pulling out, always look right! *Look right, look right, look right* became a mantra for me for a long time. I suspect the remnants of this mantra remain in my head to this day, particularly when I become a bit confused in another city. Likewise driving. After I was given an automobile on arrival, I took it out for a drive. After almost being hit by a driver as I pulled out from my driveway (*look right, look right*), I found myself coming down a steep hill, slowing as I came face to face, bonnet to bonnet, with another driver. I was thinking, *what is wrong with this person. Are they nuts?* Eventually both cars came to a dead stop, each of us staring incredulously at the other. Only then did I realize that I was on the wrong side of the road (what a surprise!). Sheepishly, and yelling apologetically as I reoriented myself to the proper side, I was met by a laugh and a wave from the other driver. I think it was the first true kindness I would meet in this new life.

And then there is the sporting world. Cricket. Looks like baseball, kind of. Hit a ball with a bat. So okay, the ball bounces off the ground before you hit it. I could deal with that. In baseball, the average number of runs scored in a major league game is in the range of six to eight. Yes, six to eight runs total for two teams. When I first read the sports page here, I saw one guy scored over 100 runs by himself! I was a bit flummoxed. How did you ever get him out? He taps the ball on the ground and just stands there. Doesn't have to run? LBW? What? I won't even get into the names of the locations on the field where players are positioned defensively. Yes, there were things to learn.

There would be many other topics to get used to here on the other side of the world, but I would adapt. The bigger problem was the so-called elephant in the room, that I had no desire to practice medicine, and I really, truly had no idea what the heck I was doing here so far from home. After about a week of stumbling around town, trying to figure out how to order in grams or kilos at the deli counter rather than in ounces or pounds, and deciphering the different brands of food that exist in the grocery store, I started to work.

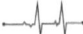

My first days are a bit of a blur, my recollections inexact. There was a morning handover meeting, when the on-call registrars 'hand over' the nighttime admissions to their team. It was here that I would reacquaint myself with being a teacher of junior doctors. It had been a long time since I had functioned as a teacher. I had forgotten how much I missed that. Those basic building blocks of knowledge and learning, however, were still there. I merely had to dust them off.

There were patients to see in the wards. Rounds to do in the Coronary Care Unit (CCU). There was no separate CCU at that time, given the small size of the department. A few beds were allocated for cardiology use in the ICU. And there was, of course, the cath lab. The place that had been a source of so many successes and failures in my life. When I arrived, the lab was being used infrequently. It had been built a few years before my arrival by predecessors who had since come and gone. Its function was to provide the equipment and space to perform diagnostic procedures. Those patients needing additional therapeutic interventions were then sent elsewhere, which meant travelling to another city – not an optimal arrangement.

More importantly, upon my arrival the lab was terribly underutilized, with minimal work being done. Essentially, diagnostic cardiac work was performed maybe one day a week by a cardiologist visiting from out of town. The staff were regularly rotated to other parts of the hospital in the absence of work being done in the lab. It was into this environment that I would step with a hope to bring the cardiac program back to life.

The cardiology department itself was, in my opinion, at least a decade behind the rest of the world. The other clinical and investigative work that the department was doing was minimal and simplistic with only two other cardiologists on staff, one of whom worked part-time. I have to say that much of this did not register with me at the time. I was too busy trying to figure out what I was supposed to be doing to be concerned about what I thought of as an underperforming department with very, very limited resources. In retrospect, to be fair, it was meant to be a basic cardiac program functioning in a general medical hospital, doing what it could. And although I felt a bit rusty, I began my work in the cath lab, doing what I was hired to do.

I had three very, very big advantages, without which the subsequent successes would never have been achieved. First, the head of the Department of Medicine was incredibly supportive. When I directly asked him what kind of work, what types of procedures he wanted me to perform in the lab, his answer was that I should do whatever I thought should be done. Simple. He left me free to make my own decisions, unfettered, allowing me the breathing space to take the department into what was then the modern world of interventional cardiology. I realize that nowadays this would not happen. There would be an endless series of committees and meetings, usually with individuals within the public service with little direct knowledge of cardiac work. And quite likely, the ultimate evolution and expansion of the cath lab, as well as the overall department of cardiology, would never come to pass. I like to think he made a good decision so many years ago to allow me that breathing space, and I hope that the thousands of patients that would follow would agree.

My second major advantage was the trainee working in the department who served as my fellow. He was far from a trainee. He had years of experience, having been trained in India and practiced for many years in the Middle East. On arrival in Australia, his qualifications as a cardiologist were not recognized by the Royal Australasian College of Physicians, and he thus had to spend two to three years in an advanced training position supervised by, well, me, along with the two other staff cardiologists. He would subsequently finish the training and join the department, becoming an integral member of our developing program. His knowledge and work ethic were a major contribution in allowing me to get my feet on the ground and shift my attention to becoming a doctor again.

The third major advantage I had, and far from the least, was the staff in the department. There is truly no way for me to express my thanks and admiration for this group, other than to acknowledge their contributions. The departmental secretary took care of me. She was forever loyal and repeatedly went beyond the call of duty. Not a day would pass that she would not stop and find me to ask if I needed anything before she left. This, in a public hospital, is unheard of. Secretarial and clerical staff are often the 'low man on the totem pole' in the hierarchy of a hospital. Yet nothing happens without them. No way could I have done what I did without her. The nursing and radiographic staff that I had inherited were … what can I say but exceptional! I was new to them and confused as hell. Yet they would follow my lead to wherever I took them. They fought the good fight in the early days when this cath lab was coming into its own. Night and day, 24 hours a day and 7 days a week, they came when I asked, and did what I asked, and held me up when, at least internally, I was falling. They were to become, in my humble opinion, one of the best cath lab staffs anywhere. The skill set was diverse, expert, and always willing to learn. A culture of excellence was being born. I have always known that without this team that I inherited upon my arrival, what happened next would never have come to pass.

And so with these three advantages, despite the loneliness, the strangeness, the isolation, the vocabulary, and the underlying fact that I did not want to be a doctor, I began my work in Tasmania.

CHAPTER 11
Finding a new home

We must be willing to get rid of the life we planned so as to have the life that is waiting for us.

— Joseph Campbell

My first week at the hospital found me scrubbed with a 56-year-old man on the table. He had been admitted into the hospital with chest pain that was classic for heart disease, and a rise in his cardiac enzymes, those proteins released by damaged cardiac muscle. The presentation was a typical one for a patient having a mild heart attack. He was brought down to the cath lab for an angiogram and discovered to have a discrete lesion (narrowing) of over 90 per cent in the proximal portion of one of the three major vessels. If you can envision the beginning or origin of an artery as point A, flowing downstream to point B, the term proximal refers to the problem being very close to point A. This physical location within the artery is extremely important. The more 'proximal' the blockage versus a 'distal' location, the more heart muscle is at risk, and thus the more dangerous it is. The obvious therapeutic approach was to intervene and place a stent into the vessel. The decision was a relatively straightforward one, even if I briefly acknowledged to myself … 'uh-oh'.

Thinking back to that moment, I knew that I was a bit 'rusty'. I had been out of the lab for over eight months, and while things were easily coming back to me, I felt nervous at the thought of performing a more complex intervention. Besides my own personal hesitancy, I was unsure about the skillset of my nurses, along with uncertainty about the equipment that was available in the hospital. Despite my reluctance about getting back into the world of medicine, now that I was here, there was no burying my head in the sand. This was the real world, and it was a real person lying there.

Then there was the logistics of it all. At that time, this was not a procedure (that word again) commonly done at this hospital, for a multitude of reasons, the primary one being the absence of a surgical backup option.

Since the advent of angioplasty of the coronary vessels, there had always been an emergency surgical option available, and only hospitals with surgical programs were performing coronary interventions. As you now know, in the early days of coronary angioplasty, complications and failures were not uncommon, and there was a time that an interventionalist could not proceed unless he was made aware that a surgical theatre was on standby, just in case. While coronary interventional procedures had evolved dramatically since the advent of stents ten years before my arrival in Tasmania, there was yet to be published data on outcomes of PCI (percutaneous coronary intervention, a term that would replace angioplasty) anywhere in the world where surgery was not available (commonly referred to as off-site PCI). It was talked about in the cardiac community, but the data was absent. And I knew of nowhere that had moved in this new direction.

Knowing all of this, I was of the opinion that it could be safely done if the cases were selected appropriately. Yet I was also new to this part of the world and was not certain as to the protocols of practice. Having seen the coronary images of the patient, I remember turning to my scrub nurse and asking her, 'What should I do?'

She asked me, 'What do you want to do?'

I said, 'Well, I would fix him!'

And she said, 'Okay, let's fix him!' Why I would accept her nod of approval to proceed as a high-level authorization only makes me giggle today. And yet that simple, almost slapstick conversation was to be my first interventional case in Tasmania. The nurses were ready. The equipment was stocked. We proceeded to a successful conclusion. And with that initial spontaneous decision, the stage was set for what was to come.

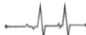

I think back often on how this evolving, and at times complex procedure, was to come to life here, in Launceston, at the end of the planet, bottom of the world. Just two people standing at the table, looking at each other, shrugging our shoulders, and saying 'Okay'. He was fixed, sent home the next day and that was that. A new era was born. And thus, the interventional program got started with me, my nursing staff, and my radiographer. No longer were patients being transferred to other locations to have interventions done. The closest hospital that was performing this procedure was approximately two hundred kilometres away.

It was a big moment for the hospital, and for the community, despite almost no one in the building being even vaguely aware of what was transpiring daily in our corner of it. Serious work, with potentially catastrophic consequences, was being performed with almost no recognition by the administration. I doubt anyone within the administration even knew what a cath lab was or what was done there, let alone would recognize that we were part of a historic undertaking. It was likely for the best, however. It has been my lived experience that the more managers within an administrative system know of something new happening, the more roadblocks are constructed.

The first whiff I had that someone was paying attention was an article that appeared in the local paper of the capital city of Tasmania, Hobart. 'Outlawed' angioplasty was being performed in the state! The program in Launceston might not be appropriate or legal! We had been in operation now for a few months when this was published. Having then read the article, I did what I would learn to do a thousand more times over the ensuing years. I did nothing. My radiographer pinned the article on the blackboard as a reminder, where it remains to this day, and we all went about getting the work done.

In today's world, this type of undertaking would never have gotten off the ground. The governance in the public system is such, that even the smallest change in protocols must meander through various committees, in the belief that their inspection of the change is required to protect the public good. Never mind what we were doing in Launceston! Patient safety is a huge topic nowadays in hospital protocols. Entire departments and governance chains have been created to protect the public good when it comes to health care. Who would argue with tha? No one would debate the need for patient safety. I would merely comment that long before the 'system' woke up to the topic, physicians were doing just that. After all, *that is the job.* Weighing risks and benefits to the patient, daily. Do no harm.

This was an historic shift in cardiac care both here and throughout the world. I believed that the best thing to do was to just keep on doing what we were doing, which was to do good work for a lot of people in the community. After two years, I would publish our interventional outcome data after the first consecutive thirteen hundred patients were completed, demonstrating results equivalent to anywhere in the world, despite the absence of on-site open-heart surgery facilities. This practice has now been taken up all over the country and the rest of the world.

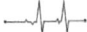

Something else was happening. Something equally profound to the work that was transpiring. I was … *happy*. I was … *feeling* again. For the patients. For the future. For a life still yet unlived. Making a difference is why many of us go into medicine to begin with. But what was happening inside me was something bordering on a resurrection. Almost a personal redemption. During those early months, my interest, my desire, my energy was returning. I was teaching. I was reading. I would attend morning handover meetings and watch and listen and teach the junior doctors the basic building blocks of cardiology. I was becoming purposeful. I was awakening from the doldrums that had consumed me for years, and the fears and worries and loneliness were subsiding. Here, at the end of the planet, I was becoming, once again, alive. The spiral that created more and more social isolation in my life was finally being severed. Fulfilling work and new relationships allowed me to see a life worth living.

FINDING A NEW HOME

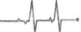

A 73-year-old woman, Joyce, arrived with a very classic patten of unstable angina. She had undergone open-heart surgery only three months previously. Given the excellent outcomes with surgery, this was a bit of a surprise, particularly given how ill she appeared. Based on well-published outcome data from bypass surgery, the likelihood of a bypass graft failure (becoming obstructed or completely occluding) in the first three months may be as high as 10 per cent or greater. Generally, these patients are asymptomatic due to a variety of flow characteristics in the arteries. But overall, the outcome of surgery is excellent. The question remained, was it excellent for Joyce.

She arrived on the table with ongoing chest pain and a low blood pressure, in the 70s. Her ECG was quite abnormal, demonstrating active ischemia, the diagnosis of something wrong being in no doubt. The angiogram demonstrated anatomy that I had never seen before, nor since. It was a convoluted map of grafts and vessels connected in ways that I found indecipherable. At that point, we managed to get the hand-sketched drawings from the surgery. These usually accompany the operative report, detailing where the bypasses were anatomically constructed. Even the drawings revealed a revascularization map that I had never seen. Reading the operative report, however, revealed that during the surgery, the left main coronary artery, feeding blood supply to the majority of the heart, was accidentally damaged. To repair this segment, surgical glue was utilized, and the left main artery was reimplanted into the aorta, followed by a series of grafts, that, once again, would not have been decipherable without the drawings.

The details at this point are less relevant than the fact that despite the unusual nature of the surgical grafts and repair work, *all* the bypasses had failed in these few months. Joyce was literally back to square one, plus some surgical glue in part of the anatomy that was, to say, unusual.

This complex anatomy was beyond a stenting strategy. Joyce was acutely ill, with chest pain and hypotension. A balloon pump was inserted to aid in coronary flow, the only recourse left but to send her back for a re-do operation only months since her last surgery.

I hate to say that having just moved from an extremely litigious country where medical malpractice claims are a part of daily life, my first thought was: *This is absolutely going to go to court. I can hear them calling the lawyers now.* But I was not in the US. Having stabilized her on the table, I turned to Joyce to explain that the first surgery had utterly failed. She would need to be sent back to the surgeon as an emergency for another operation. And we were calling the transport paramedics to come shortly for her. Much to my surprise, and frankly, my amazement, she looked at me and simply said, 'Well, I know that they did the best they could do.' Not what I was expecting. Such decency.

This is not an easy business and bad things do happen. But she accepted her fate with a degree of equanimity that frankly, I do not know that I possess. It was a reminder that I was in a very different place in the world from the one I had left.

With that, Joyce was sent out of town for another operation. Unfortunately, the surgeon turned her down due to the complications of her first surgery, and she would go on to die suddenly, three days later in hospital, after attempts were made by others to fix her with stents. Everyone was doing the best that they could do. It was a terrible outcome in a woman who clearly was gentle and decent.

These stories never leave you.

Prior to these new beginnings, and before I transplanted myself to the other side of the world, I was involved in a case with a woman in her late forties who was found to have moderate cardiac dysfunction on ultrasound and was subsequently diagnosed with multi-vessel coronary disease. The solution was clearly open-heart surgery. She was discharged home for outpatient elective surgery in the weeks ahead. Up until the diagnosis, she was almost completely asymptomatic. This was nearly an accidental discovery, despite the very real danger it would pose if left untreated. The following week she presented to the hospital with her first bout of chest pain, ever. It is not uncommon for patients to begin to get pain once they know there is something wrong! She was quite stable, with no significant consequence to this hospitalization, other than having her surgery moved up on the list while she was an inpatient. Everything went fine and discharge occurred five days post-op.

A few months later, I received notification that I was being sued. She claimed that she had suffered further heart damage while waiting for her elective surgery. She had not. Her heart had already suffered damage before I had ever met her. No further cardiac injury occurred during this new admission. Nevertheless, I was being sued for inappropriate delay in treatment.

I would subsequently learn that this woman had substance abuse problems, was unemployed, and legally responsible for supporting her children. Whether these social issues may have had any bearing on the pursuit of this case remains an unknown, but my suspicions of a pay day were certainly there. Naturally, once you are sued, the barrage of paperwork and lawyer appointments begins, culminating in a deposition, sworn testimony in the presence of lawyers representing both yourself and the suing party.

This was not my first deposition, but nonetheless, a process that one must be prepared for since this information is used at the time of trial. I never found out what transpired with the case. By the time it came around for final legal discussion with her attorney and my malpractice lawyer, I had left the country. I did not care about the outcome. I was personally disgusted with it all. And now I was gone. Most of these cases are settled out of court by malpractice insurers to save on legal fees.

What was striking for me was the juxtaposition of this 'malpractice' case and the preceding story of Joyce. The nature of the 'insult' and the magnitude of the response. In the case of Joyce, I relate a story of a woman who had endured a terrible outcome, ultimately paying with her life. All she had to offer me was her thanks for doing the best we could do. On the other, was a woman who had nothing inappropriate happen during the course of her treatment, but sensing an opportunity, unleashed the legal system to rectify a 'wrong' that was non-existent. For me, these two stories just about summed up my feelings at that time. This latter encounter was the world I had left. The former, well … it speaks for itself.

I didn't know it then, but my life was about to change.

CHAPTER 12
Teacher

I touch the future. I teach.

— Christa McAuliffe

I arrived in Tasmania knowing no one. Yet during those early months following my arrival, I was shown generosity and kindness by patients and by staff. It was a significant change for me. Isolation was seemingly a thing of the past and slowly, very slowly, I was witness to the creation of a 'community' in which I was a part. The professional challenges were different. The environment was different. The health system itself was different. I saw a future where I could fulfill those naïve thoughts of decades ago … that I could make a difference in the world …

It was my choice to come to this island state and make it my home. I arrived in a fog, clueless as to what would come next. Those first three months were extended to six. I woke up from a very dark place and saw into a future. What I wished to do, what drove me to ultimately move across the ocean, was build something new. To establish a cardiology program that would persist beyond my time. I saw the opportunity, and the need. It was far from only an unselfish motivation, however. For in the making of that new 'thing', I was also making a new me. A better me. If it was my sons that kept me alive during many of the darkest days of my life, then Tasmania would be the place where I could put that saved life to a greater use.

First, it would entail providing a clinical service in the public hospital that was sorely lacking. Hopefully, a better and more complete service. That was step one. Step two was to expand my teaching role. It is that part of my career where I have felt the most satisfaction and the most enjoyment. Once the clinical program was up and running, this next step entailed developing a training program for those wishing to make cardiology their lifelong work. To touch the future.

General cardiology is the bedrock from which to begin such training. Without the foundation of this underpinning knowledge, the more complex subsequent building blocks are far more likely to crumble with time. To become a general cardiologist, three years are given to learn the basics of knowledge and practice the technical skills required. These are not easy years. It is a busy clinical service during the day, and a sleepless one at night. In Launceston, the workload was relentless. And while the overall supervision of the trainees in general would fall to me along with my few colleagues, it was the teaching in the cath lab that was clearly what I was most interested in.

So, with this in mind, our small group of what was now one full-time and two part-time general cardiologists, along with me as the sole interventionalist, created a new teaching program. It was initially to be accredited for one year, then two, and eventually three years – the time frame required by the Royal College of Physicians to achieve one's fellowship in Cardiology. During this early period in the program, I was the sole practitioner on call for emergency procedures, 24 hours a day, 7 days a week. To attain the hoped-for goal of becoming a three-year training program was a slow and gradual process that stretched over five years, but it was, and remains, an astonishing accomplishment for a hospital located in what is referred to as one of the *regions* of Australia, that is, a non-metropolitan centre (already at the bottom of the planet, at the end of the world).

With the growth of the teaching program, of course, new responsibilities arose. Those responsibilities included making sure your trainees didn't cause serious harm to the patient! It can be a tightrope you walk as a supervisor in the cath lab. Teaching invasive skills requires handing over the equipment to another, gradually teaching them how to use the tools. As the trainee progresses, the nature of the techniques becomes more subtle and more dangerous. Yet you must let them progress. They, too, are 'practicing' medicine. But that means giving them 'enough rope to hang themselves', without hanging the patient with it!

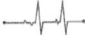

First thing Monday morning, my advanced trainee (AT), who was now in his second year, was starting the first case of the week. A simple and straightforward (beware!) diagnostic angiogram, something he had done over five hundred times by then. I was sitting at my desk in the cath lab, keeping an eye on the procedure, while I was looking over the work coming up for the rest of the day. (At this stage of training, scrubbing alongside your AT is not required for all cases. Their experience is considerable by this point.)

Vascular access was complete, and the AT began to take his first images. Following the first dye injection, I was asked to take a look at this first angiographic picture, which showed the injected dye sitting in the patient's left main coronary, not going anywhere. Normally the contrast dye immediately washes out of the vessel as blood continues to traverse the artery. This dye was going nowhere. If the dye is not moving, neither is the blood flow! It appeared that no one else in the room fully appreciated what that meant. But I did. And it was not good.

I immediately jumped up, threw on my lead apron, and began ordering the equipment that was now necessary, the tools now needed. The first image taken clearly demonstrated that the AT had inadvertently torn or dissected the left main. Catastrophe was around the corner. Without a fix, probable death. This complication, although not common, can happen to anyone. Knowing what to do about it is another matter. These are the moments when I, only half-jokingly, say to myself and my trainees, 'Test your own sphincter tone.'

After the quick insertion of another catheter, I was fortunate to find my way through the dissected vessel, which now had not only dissected the left main artery but had then found dual false pathways into both the anterior descending and circumflex artery (so-called 'bifurcation'). Using small and flexible wires, I felt my way as much as I visually watched the wires under x-ray guidance, negotiate through these dissected segments. But once the wires were in the right place, it was a matter of working quickly to re-establish blood flow to both arterial distributions and put stents in at multiple sites to 'tack up' the torn wall. On paper it's pretty easy, but in the real world, when patients are having chest pain, the ECG showing major changes, and the blood pressure readings are falling, it can be a nightmare. These are some of the days, I have often commented to my fellows, that you are better off being lucky than good. I like to think that skill begets the good luck, but enough of that.

The patient did fine and was discharged two days later with this complication thoroughly discussed and explained. There were no untoward consequences. Never withhold the truth about complications. Never. I teach my ATs the same.

The other casualty of this event was my AT. That early in training, particularly if you have never seen such a complication, such an occurrence can be a crushing blow. One day you think it's all simple, with success achieved on a regular basis, and the next you become fearful to do ... anything. You know that you literally almost killed the patient. It is quite sobering. I gave him enough rope ... The patient was fine. My AT would go on to finish his basic training, begin training further, and now works as an interventional cardiologist. He clearly overcame the fear that is generated by such a life-endangering event. But I would bet my life that he has never forgotten that single angiographic injection, the image, nor the lessons learned on that day.

Supervising trainees was to become a major and important aspect of my work in the ensuing years. Teaching, watching, gauging situations, knowing when to step in and take over and when to give the AT some space. I have done it thousands of times, and every situation is different. It may be something as simple as trying to find an artery to access, finding the right catheter that fits. Maybe it's getting a better angle on a picture to see what you are looking for or just manoeuvring the catheter through diseased vessels before reaching the heart. I have watched the ATs spend fifteen minutes or more attempting a manoeuvre that I would step in and perform in seconds. You have to give them time. It's a learning curve. It all requires technical skills. But in truth, alongside technique, this endeavour, putting devices inside the heart, really is a thinking man's game. When things go smoothly, it seems that anyone can do it. If it doesn't, then whoever is standing there needs to problem solve. Fast. Usually, the problem is one that can be solved. Sometimes it is not.

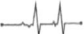

Following a 'straightforward' angiogram, a 68-year-old woman was found to have a focal blockage in a major artery. My AT was quite advanced at the time, and so I asked him to access the coronary artery with a guiding catheter in preparation for a PCI to the vessel. While he was performing this relatively routine task, the patient had some slight chest pain. A little test injection showed that the catheter was not in the coronary artery yet, but there was a disturbing appearance of the aorta itself.

I stepped in and exchanged the catheter for a pigtail catheter, so called for its shape, and did an injection into the root of the aorta. Lo and behold, due to the manipulation of the guiding catheter in the hands of the AT, the patient's aorta had acquired a catheter-induced, *ENORMOUS* dissection, creating a huge flap pulsating with the blood flow. Accompanying this very extensive dissection, she developed a massive amount of regurgitant, or leaking flow through her aortic valve. This can occur when the aorta dissects right down to its root origins. This cannot be fixed in a cath lab. The situation, stable moments ago, had now turned into a surgical emergency. I was amazed at how stable she was, despite both a massive aortic dissection and severe aortic insufficiency, but it didn't change the fact that we had to fly her out ASAP for surgery that day.

Fortunately, she remained stable, had her operation, and lived to fight another day. My AT was profoundly shaken. A routine manoeuvre had resulted in a near-catastrophic event. I was standing right beside him, but there was nothing for me to do to fix the patient. This was a problem not 'solvable' in the cath lab. In this case, it was making the diagnosis quickly, and deciding the next move, not pretending to yourself that it is not happening. It is guaranteed that the AT has not forgotten.

This was a far cry from what I had witnessed a few years earlier by a junior colleague, a newly trained interventionalist from another institution in his first consultancy role. I happened to walk into the lab where there was much commotion going on. During the set-up for a PCI on a male patient, yet again the origin of the coronary vessel had become dissected. In this case, rather than creating a small linear flap that could be fixed with a stent, the dissection had spiralled its way down the entire length of the artery and was as complex a dissection as I had ever seen. It was impossible to tell the true lumen, or opening, apart from the false one created by this tear. In addition, the dissection extended out the coronary into the aorta, up the aorta towards the arteries supplying the brain, around the aortic arch, and subsequently extended down his entire thorax passing the renal arteries, which are situated mid-way to the legs. I have seen many dissections. This was the worst. You literally could not tell where normal artery was. This was a *HUGE* dissection. It could not be repaired in the cath lab.

More importantly, even if by some miracle the operator was able to repair the coronary vessel, the patient would need an operation to repair the aorta anyway. And yet, my colleague had been spending the hour trying to fix the spiral dissection in the coronary artery, with almost no hope of success. There was no point in spending the time. He was looking at the 'tree' without seeing the 'forest'. Emergency surgery was indicated. He was fortunate that despite a massive complication, the patient was stable. That, or unbelievably stoic. He did not complain. I convinced my colleague to stop what he was doing and get an ambulance for transport. Seniority has its advantages.

The lesson here is that you cannot deny what is happening in this business. Make the diagnosis, consider what needs to be done, and do it. There is much to say about the kind of complications I have witnessed, and it is the recurring issue in these stories. They happen, and not infrequently. What separates the proverbial men from the boys, is knowing what to do next.

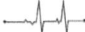

As a supervisor and senior operator, you become the 'bail out' for problems. As I have tried to illustrate, some days you win, some you lose. But it's the patient safety that is of the utmost importance.

I was called to a case that had started as a simple PCI (once again, 'simple': be wary) when all things took a turn for the worse. Following the initial ballooning of the arterial plaque, the wire used to maintain access into the coronary artery was inadvertently pulled out. At that point the patient started to get severe chest pain. A test injection showed what had been a patent artery was now completely occluded following the trauma of the balloon inflation. The operator was desperately trying to open the artery again but could not find the true lumen of the vessel with the wire. A case that was less than ten minutes from completion had now turned into, for want of other words, a mess.

After numerous attempts to rescue the vessel had been made, I was called as the emergency backup guy. I was not in the building. I was in the town swimming pool being tapped on the head by a lifeguard as I was making my turn at the wall, being summoned to an emergency call from the hospital. One of my nurses had known where to find me. Once I got the message, I was off to the races. You know what it's like trying to get dressed quickly when you are wet? If you don't, give it a try. Fortunately, the hospital is literally a five-minute drive, and I got there fairly quickly, only to find a room packed with doctors and nurses and the patient moaning in pain, with her ECG clearly showing an evolving heart attack due to the loss of this major vessel.

Once in the room, I was able to re-establish flow within minutes and fix the problem. It was then that the nurses began to think that I could fix anything. Far from it. Maybe it was just another lucky day for me. And, more importantly, for the patient, who would be discharged home without any heart damage two days later.

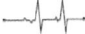

Now I found myself training new cardiologists, at the highest technical level, in this regional hospital with no surgery on site. As the program grew and the trainee numbers grew, I established a fellowship in Interventional Cardiology. I cannot begin to tell you how extraordinarily unusual it was, and is, to have such a fellowship program in a regional hospital in Australia. It was unprecedented at the time. The training was for those who had finished their three years in general cardiology and wanted to effectively do what I was doing. They each wanted to become an interventionalist. Another two to three years and they would be ready. It is such a long haul to get through the training; so many sleepless nights; so many phone calls. So much responsibility to live up to in order to achieve their goal.

The department invented some creative funding for the position. For a relatively small hospital, the volume of patients was large, and I was determined to begin teaching at this level. Allowing trainees to move to this next phase was a new test for me. Allowing them to take images of the heart is one thing. To train them in the manipulation of wires, balloons, stents and other ancillary equipment inside the beating heart was yet another. We were moving into more dangerous territory as the demands of the work were intensifying and the risks to the patients were escalating. And yet, it was the best work I have ever done, and the most rewarding teaching I have ever participated in. To teach someone to do intracardiac interventions is a slow, arduous task, but when they come out of the other end as a skilled operator, it is transformative.

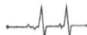

A young woman in her thirties was transferred from Emergency to the cath lab late on a Friday evening with the possible diagnosis of cardiac tamponade (a condition you have already heard much about).

My fellow had called me from Emergency that evening with the patient's history and a cardiac ultrasound that was suspicious, but not diagnostic of tamponade. I did not want this case to sit over the weekend without a diagnosis, and so I decided to move forward for a definitive diagnostic study, and treatment if needed. It was not a straightforward decision, but given the possible consequence of a delay or missed opportunity for treatment, it seemed reasonable to proceed that evening. I had my fellow notify the call team, and the patient was taken to the lab.

As I have often done in these particular cases, I used a right heart catheter to quantify the necessary haemodynamics to support or dismiss the diagnosis. As soon as intracardiac pressures were measured, however, the diagnosis of tamponade was clear cut. A pericardiocentesis was required.

I looked at my fellow, who had yet to perform one, but had scrubbed in and observed many others. It was now his turn. 'See one, do one, teach one', an old adage, may be a bit simplistic. But it really was his turn.

It was just at that moment, literally, that the patient crashed abruptly. Her BP, stable only minutes ago, had plummeted, and she became severely agitated.

My fellow, a man I have trained for the preceding three years, is one of the good ones. I tell him to step into the primary operator's position at the table, look at him, and ask, 'Are you ready to do this?'

Without hesitation he answers, 'Yes,' all the while quickly prepping the patient's chest. I am feeling my sphincter tone being tested yet again as I watch him slide the needle under her sternum, searching for the fluid in the pericardial sac. This is an emergency.

I have always been a bit agitated teaching this technique, given what I have seen happen in the past. I am ready to move him aside within seconds if success is not swiftly achieved. My confidence in him is quickly vindicated as yellow fluid is aspirated into the syringe and a drainage catheter is advanced into position. The young woman on the table will leave the hospital days later. If we had not brought her to the lab on this Friday evening, if we had elected to 'watch her' on the wards, I seriously doubt she would have survived. The crash happened so suddenly. Under intense pressure, my fellow has likely saved his first life. For me, training young minds to do this: what a privilege.

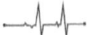

This case was a great saving of life. I would hope things always go so well. It is not the way it always plays out. One of my other fellows was doing a simple (that word again) PCI to one artery, when following ballooning of the vessel, he inadvertently removed the wire holding the artery open before deploying a stent. The artery occluded. This time, despite my best efforts, I could not restore flow. I simply could not find my way back through this now suddenly occluded vessel. The BP of the patient had remained stable but the ECG changes on the monitor were clearly consistent with an abrupt coronary occlusion.

One reaches a point during these 'rescue' procedures, trying to fix a complication that has just been created, where the risks of continuing potentially outweigh the risks of stopping. There is no rule book for this. These kinds of decisions are based almost solely on experience, that probability equation that you acquire over time. You guess. I elected to stop the case after a prolonged attempt at rescue. The patient had a heart attack, and three days later died of renal failure. What appeared easy, was not. The problem was created by simple human error. And on this occasion, I failed to make it better. Despite what the nurses had come to believe, I could not fix everything. Those failures have never left me; every case in which I have failed has never been forgotten.

While in the middle of a difficult case one day, I turned around to lean on the scrub table trying to figure out what to do next. I looked up at the circulating nurse, shaking my head from side to side, the visual cue that I was in trouble. She just looked at me and said, 'Don't worry, you always know what to do.'

I got through that case, but I thought, *if only your statement was always true.*

I can understand why teachers often love what they do. All jobs have a bit of a grind to them, where the day-to-day is just that, a grind. But when you see the light brighten over a student, when you know that you have given that student the gift of knowledge or experience, maybe even a light-bulb moment, the satisfaction is truly affirming. It has been rewarding to see my own knowledge base grow through the years, and my technical skills getting better with age. Yet it's the teaching that I find has carried me over time.

I was at the cath table one day, explaining to my fellow what my approach was going to be, showing him how to shape the wires we were using in a more complex bifurcation lesion. He turned to me and said, 'Doesn't seem fair that what has taken you thirty years to learn, you teach me in ten minutes.'

I must admit I had never thought of it that way! From the early years of PCI, when balloons were the sole tool of the trade and minimal drugs were available, I have literally been self-taught the rest of the time. I have had other interventionalists visit our lab, serving as proctors for non-coronary work, expanding my repertoire of intracardiac techniques. But in coronary interventions, I have learned almost all on my own. As each new generation of equipment and techniques came into being, I had to learn to use them with little assistance. Here I was now, giving my fellow a life's experience, acquired through lots of trial and error, in a few minutes of teaching. A few moments passed as I contemplated his comment. I admit that I did not like it! None of it, on face value, seemed fair! Such selfish thoughts. But I was quick to acknowledge that we all stand on the shoulders of those who came before us, and we are all the beneficiaries of their life work. This was just the passing down of another generation of knowledge. I liked my fellow. He was a good guy with excellent skills. It was not lost on him. This was what I had helped create. It was my best work.

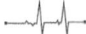

I was reasonably athletic as a child. Not great. Not terrible. As I related in an earlier chapter, my childhood was full of play. It is what I lived for.

One of the rare organized athletic activities available in the Bronx was Little League baseball. You would wear a baseball hat and a real-looking professional-style uniform with the name of your team on the back. You got to play on a real grass baseball field, those few scattered around our neighbourhood, which outside of Little League were off limits to us. Just like the big time. Little League starts around the time you are nine years old and moves on over the next four or five years, and even beyond for those with a real aptitude and desire to play at a higher level.

One year we were playing in the 'World Series'. A bit of a misnomer, but within the confines of the local league, this is the final. By then, I was a decent player and tasked with playing shortstop, a pivotal position in the infield.

We are out in the field, the last inning, with the opponents' tying run on third base when the next batter steps up to the plate. The coach is exhorting everyone to get ready to make the play. It is a tense moment for us. There are two outs and the next at bat could determine the winner of the game.

I am crouched in position, pounding my glove while chattering in the infield to the pitcher, encouraging him on. 'Let's get this guy out. Strike him out! We got this guy.' Yet inside my head, filled with the excitement of the possible win, the glory that this would bring, I am saying to the deaf world, the world that cannot hear me, 'Please, don't hit the ball to me!'

You see, I didn't want the ball. I didn't want to be the hero. Well, yeah, I did, but I was far more afraid of not making the play. Of being the failure. And so I didn't want that ball! 'Please don't hit the ball to me!!' The fear of a child – of all men and women who don't want the ball.

I am grown now. I have seen the worst things happen in my profession and I have been nearly broken many times over the years. But now I have merged experience with skill and knowledge, and I teach others, I hope, the same. I have stepped in often to bail out others. I have tackled the most complex cases. It took a long time. Now, when things are tough, when decisions are difficult, when technical problems arise, *now*, I want the ball. Now, '*Gimme the ball!*'

CHAPTER 13
Reputation

Character is like a tree, and reputation like its shadow. The shadow is what we think of it; the tree is the real thing.

— Abraham Lincoln

In 1979, the movie *Being There*, starring Peter Sellers, was released. One of my favourites, seen at a time when I was still trying to make heads or tails of the world. Sellers portrays a simple-minded man named Chance, who has spent his entire life tending to the sequestered gardens of an elderly wealthy benefactor in the midst of Washington DC. When the old man passes away, the bank descends upon the property and Chance is forced to leave the only place he has known as home, with no knowledge of the outside world other than what he has seen on TV. Wearing the old man's well-tailored, if out-of-style suits taken from the attic, Chance is accidentally struck by a passing car of a wealthy woman portrayed by Shirley MacLaine. She immediately must tend to his injuries and mistakes his name, Chance the gardener, for Chauncey Gardiner. After driving him with his injuries to her home, her husband, a friend of the President of the USA, is taken by 'Chauncey', thinking him a wealthy businessman based on his attire. His simple, naive utterances are thought to be deep meaningful interpretations of world events. When later asked about his opinion of the world economic situation, his comments about the changes of weather and how it will affect growth in the garden are thought to be cryptic comments on the positive state of the economy. Fortunes rise and fall on the musings of a naïve and innocent gardener. Before you know it, he is someone everyone is listening to, including the president. The utterances of a simpleton thought to be a genius. I won't relate the entire tale, no spoiler alert here, but I hope you get my drift. An allegorical tale of how reputation may grow from … nothing. Great movie.

It had me thinking though, what is the basis of a reputation, and what does it take to have a good one? How does one gain prestige, credibility, or recognition, be it from peers or the general public? Is it earned? If so, how? What does it take to lose it, assuming you ever gain it? Should you trust it? I have been puzzled with these questions for many years, if not equally vexed with some of the answers that I have seen. I write about the field of medicine, but these questions are equally valid in all fields of endeavour.

One evening, I was out having dinner at a small Korean restaurant in town with some friends who were in the restaurant business. I have always been impressed by what my friends have built in their professional career. Starting with a simple sandwich shop, they would ultimately go on to establish a 5-star, award-winning restaurant. A second restaurant would follow, helping a host of other chefs and employees with their own budding careers, along with other business ventures. All this from a simple sandwich shop. From where I was sitting, this was a remarkable feat. In a business with crazy hours and a high rate of failure, they had succeeded and had earned my respect. And my friendship. Their reputation would seem to have been earned.

So here I was having dinner with these good friends when a man approached the table and asked to shake my hand. As I stood, he reminded me that I had saved his life a few years previously, and he simply wished to say thanks for what I had done for him. I asked his name, given there was no way I could remember this very specific 'case', and thanked him for the compliment he paid me and the warmth he exhibited. It is always a bit uncomfortable to be thanked for such a thing without being able to remember any details. Uncomfortable, and sometimes embarrassing. Nevertheless, justifiable. The number of patients dealt with, even in the relatively short time of a week, can be overwhelming, and many, many details are lost over the years, at least for me.

We chatted for a few minutes, with a few jokes thrown in, and he then left the restaurant. I sat back down, and looked at my friend, who stared at me with a somewhat curious, smiling face. His father-in-law was a paediatric surgeon. He was familiar with this kind of interaction, watching previous patients coming up and thanking his father-in-law for things he had done years before. But that smile on his face. I really didn't know what it meant, but I felt that he recognized in me something new. At that moment, I felt that at least with him, my reputation had grown.

Being validated by someone you respect. Is that how one does it? Gain a good reputation? I remember the incident quite clearly because for me, this was a new feeling. In my 'old life', I probably did not deserve this kind of recognition. It was only in this latter half of my career that this form of acknowledgement came my way. And truthfully? I am not certain that I have ever been entirely comfortable with it.

Similarly, a year earlier, I was at the travel agency booking a flight to who knows where and chatting with the travel agent. A woman came up to me, asking me if I was … me, and when I said that I was, she put her arms around me and gave me a hug. 'Thank you again,' she said, 'for saving my life,' – which had been three years earlier. Once again, I asked her name, told a few jokes to disguise my lapse in memory, and thanked her for coming up to me and letting me know she was well. I really enjoy those moments. Who wouldn't?

I turned back to the travel agent, who by the way, was also a previous patient of mine, to find him smiling, then chuckling. He had been where she had been. Her public gratitude towards me affirmed an opinion that was likely already formed by him. Again, it felt (to me) as if my reputation was growing. So, is that how it comes about? Reinforcement by multiple sources? Reputation: not a physical reality. Not tangible. Yet quite real in its effects.

I have had a love-hate relationship with this subject for many years. For I have been on both sides of it. One day lauded for excellence, the next being questioned in a deposition as to why a bad outcome occurred. I have been the heroic winner. I have been the broken loser.

Does a good reputation really mean you are good and skilled at what you do? Let's stick with the medical profession for now. It is, after all, what I know. Countless patients over many, many years have remarked to me how good their general practitioner is, or said that the specialist they saw was the best in the area. Only rarely have I been told the opposite. It happens, but not nearly as often as the good stuff. I don't doubt that thinking your doctor is terrific is very reassuring. That's a nice thing, but is everybody really that good? How is that measured? Is everyone a platinum five-star jubilee doctor?

Being a physician, just having the diploma, already seems to confer a certain status. A certain trustworthiness. On the Ipsos Global Trustworthiness Ranking 2024, doctors are ranked at the top of the list (note that politicians are the lowest). Within the medical profession, nurses are ranked even higher, likely reflecting the personal care they provide to patients when they are at their neediest. Clearly, this is a job that comes with a certain advantage if one is in fact seeking gratitude and approval in life. It is almost 'built in' the day you graduate. So, what else do you have to do besides get past the exams?

Once, long ago, I was asked by a woman if I knew her son, a cardiologist in Atlanta, Georgia. I privately wondered why she would think I would know of her son who was living over a thousand miles from me. I answered her that I did not. She went on to tell me how well her son was regarded, and that naturally, he was at the top of his field: a very respected and successful man and doctor. She clearly loved her son and was immensely proud of what he was doing. That's a nice thing. Nevertheless, reputation has its limits. In my world, he was just another guy.

See, that's the thing. Many of these 'best' specialists in whatever, and 'great' general so and so's, are, for me, just another guy. No five star ratings. No platinum awards. Let's face it, on a bell-shaped curve, most people are kind of in the middle … average. So how are so many of them so 'great'?

It is not uncommon that a certain status in the medical community is built on something other than knowledge or skill. Most of us like to think that these two things, skill and knowledge, would or should be prerequisites to earning positive recognition.

Yet, it is not so.

A solid reputation may be based on the virtue of really caring for the patient. By itself, caring for the patients is an important feature of all branches of medical practice. Maybe the most important. And being able to communicate this commitment to the patient is, in itself, a useful tool for promoting good health. Yet within this cohort of caring doctors are those who do not necessarily have good skills, or up-to-date knowledge. Lacking knowledge and expertise, empathy is substituted. Some choose to investigate everything. Batteries of tests are ordered without hesitation. X-rays, CT scans, blood work, ultrasounds. It's a shotgun approach. Shoot wide and hope that you hit something. Get enough tests, and you might find something. The patient simply concludes that the doctor really cares and doesn't want to miss anything important.

This, unfortunately, can easily cover up a lack of clinical insight, relying on frequent testing in the hope of diagnosing everything, or indeed anything. This is not a blanket condemnation. I would infinitely rather have investigations done for a problem that a doctor is uncertain of, or be referred to someone with a greater expertise. But on the other hand, ordering tests and being 'nice' are not the factors, the reasons, the rationales, to bestow on someone a good reputation. At least not for me.

I knew a GP in the US who would see his patients, without fail, every two weeks in the office. He was known in the medical community as one who was very, very out of touch with advances in medicine, having failed to maintain any continuing medical education. He had a small practice. The patients thought he was a caring doctor because he would see them so frequently, checking their blood pressure, weight, et cetera; ordering blood work several times a year. They really liked him. Yet it was obvious to anyone in the business, the real reason for seeing the patients so frequently was that it was the only way he could fill up his office appointments! Maybe a shock to some, but this, after all, is a business. Perhaps not the typical business, but a business nevertheless.

Another means of gaining status and prestige is to join a large and successful practice. If you appear, or even are, by some measure 'successful', patients assume that excellence must reside in the premises. How easily we equate business success with competence. It simply is not true. Just because an athlete can throw a ball better than anyone on the planet, does not bestow upon him expertise on shaving cream or car rentals. Equally, a successful business model does not automatically translate into excellence in health care. Yet even medical businesses pursue this via advertising, sponsorships, and social media. Before I left the US, I would see surgical practices advertising on the back of public buses. Surgical subspecialists with billboards to see while driving on the highway! Acquiring a good reputation as a physician should be based on more than slick marketing and a longer waiting time to be seen. Yet I have seen this over and over again within my professional life, and within my own specialty. The craving for recognition. For with that being bestowed, you must be one of the special ones.

Stories abound of doctors who spend more time on the computer than looking at patients. An exquisitely designed office with state-of-the-art systems does not, and should not, confuse the patient as to how good the doctor is at their work. I had a patient who told me of how a cardiologist who had previously been her doctor would walk into the room and stand, holding onto the doorknob. No sitting. Body language to let her know that this would be a quick chat. Big practice. Nice office. Well known in the community. If your doctor doesn't let go of the doorknob when they walk in, think twice before giving a 5-star rating.

More than a decade ago, I was invited to give a dinner talk at a national interventional cardiology conference. The topic was mine to choose, but I was asked to speak about something other than pure medicine. Something that would add a bit more 'spice' to the weekend. I never knew why I was asked. Maybe because I had come from another country; maybe I was seen as someone older with a different life experience – I really don't know. But I accepted and considered my options.

After a week, I chose to speak on a topic I had become intimately acquainted with: how I had come to deal with failure. The talk centred on the failures of my professional life – the poor outcomes I had both witnessed and created. Some of those stories are recalled in these pages. It wasn't so much about the medical part. It was about how to deal with it all.

I don't think I have a particular expertise on this subject, or some great secret that I could share. Everyone learns to deal with it in their own way. But for me, the only way I ultimately could get through the moments of feeling like I was the failure, carrying the guilt and shame for years to come, was to let go of the exact opposite. I had to let go of feeling like the hero. Let go of thinking my successes made me 'special'. They are merely different sides of the same coin. When you flip this coin, you are either the winner or loser. Without the coin, you are neither. For one who wanted to be like my childhood superheroes, there was much to learn. I had to discover that in a line of work where bad things happened no matter how good you were, the goal was to be honest, skilled, and ready. Both the motivation and the decision-making to do the work had to be honestly arrived at. Skills needed to be acquired and practiced. Complications needed to be prepared for. If I could meet these criteria – honesty, skill, preparedness – then whatever the outcome, I would accept it. Who doesn't aspire to good outcomes? But there is a vast difference in wanting good outcomes and wanting good reputations. Thinking of one's reputation, as I had done many decades ago when I first began this journey, needed to be set aside if I would ever be able to live with the bad outcomes.

Anyway, it was a great talk, maybe my best ever. Even years later, those who were there remembered it. I was just thrilled to get through it. I was extraordinarily nervous, working without a script, microphone in hand, exposing myself mostly to strangers, sharing some of my most painful moments. There was something cleansing about that day. It was a turnaround point to publicly express the emotional turmoil that I had lived with created by this work, this profession, and be greeted afterwards by an audience who shared the same issues of dealing with failure. No matter what walk of life chosen. I was pleased, gratified, and strengthened by the experience.

I am happy when patients think I am the guy to come see. When someone has told them I am 'the man'. I have felt, and still feel, honoured to be thought of in a good way. But much like feeling that you're a hero or a failure, reputation can be a fleeting thing. All you can do is put your head down and do the good work for the good reasons. If you can do that, well, that's about as good as it gets.

I remember that young intern who stood in the elevator with a stethoscope around his neck, wearing his beeper, watching the passengers making room as I stepped in. Wanting the attention and the rewards that would follow. Having patients think highly of you, having 'standing' in the community, is infinitely better than being thought of as no more than average. This is undeniably true. But in this business, you are only as good as your last case. Then it's on to the next. A busy day has seen me with over a dozen patients on the table, each outcome as important as the last.

When truly earned, honour and distinction often taken a lifetime to build. Equally, it can take moments to destroy. We have seen this playing out frequently in these days of social media, particularly focused on the famous or the wealthy, sometimes the politically connected. Anyone with a spotlight on them can be taken down far quicker than it took for them to be built up. I've encountered both in my professional life: those who would throw me under the bus, and those who would hug me in a travel agency.

It is a simple lesson to all. It took a mere thirty years of practice for me to figure it out. If you want to feel the highs of being the hero, of gaining the 'best' reputation, you'd better be prepared for feeling the misery of being the failure.

CHAPTER 14

On call

Medicine is a jealous mistress.

— William Osler

The phone is ringing. It is 2:00 a.m. It's the hospital operator saying that the ICU is on the line. The operator asks if I can take the call. Naturally, I agree. Wait … in truth, there is absolutely nothing natural about any of this. Being woken in the middle of the night by phone calls is not what I look forward to. But take it I do. A moment later I am connected to a registrar talking me through the events of a patient already admitted, now having severe chest pain while in the ICU. As he is relating the details of the admission, I can hear lots of commotion in the background with the voice of the senior staff yelling out, 'Dr Herman, please just come in …' That is enough for me to hear. I know the voice, and I know it's time. I swing my legs out of bed, and for the umpteenth time find my clothes waiting for me on the floor. After so many times of being called to go to an emergency during the sleeping hours, I realized it was just easier to undress and leave my clothing lying there. Think of it as emergency wardrobe efficiency.

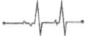

Being on call. Unless you have done this countless times, it is difficult to imagine what it is like to be tethered to your job in this way. As an interventionalist, it is more than just 'being available'. It is being available to leave wherever you are – whether that's out to dinner, at a movie theatre, home with the family, at a friend's home, the swimming pool, or the comfort of bed – get to the hospital, and arrive to emergencies that are *extremely* time sensitive.

There is an adage in interventional cardiology that time is muscle. For a patient having a large heart attack, this is exceptionally true. The quicker one can re-establish flow to an occluded artery, the more cardiac muscle tissue can be saved. Guidelines throughout the world's medical literature, published and updated over many years, all support the principle that time delays matter when it comes to heart muscle preservation. Being on call in cardiac emergencies is not just taking phone calls or even being called in to work, but being physically available to arrive at the hospital with minimal delay in order to alter the course of a major cardiac event. Doing this kind of on-call, for decades, affects almost every aspect of one's life that one can imagine.

On call includes nights, weekends, holidays and evenings after work. Anytime. Most people are aware that doctors take calls after hours. Taking phone calls and managing patient problems twenty-four hours a day can be taxing and draining, particularly when already working full days. Take that and add on what is required in this kind of on call. This is at another level. It is not a normal existence. How do you construct a normal life when your availability appears to be – no, not appears to be, but *must* be a constant? Can you go out to dinner? Do you have company over to the house? Do you go for a swim, or to the gym, or go for a run? There are constant compromises and planning required to be on call. And this is to last a professional lifetime.

When I was living in the US, before my move to Tasmania, I had spent over a decade taking call 180 days a year. Half my life was committed around the clock to my work life. It was not enjoyable, but it was what I accepted. With my initial arrival in Tasmania (now, as I write, over two decades ago), I found myself in a scenario, one that I created, of being available all hours of the day, every day. With an opportunity to build a program sorely needed in this part of Tasmania, I had accepted that for true emergencies, I would always be there: 24 hours a day, 7 days a week, 365 days a year. I look back on that decision with mixed thoughts and feelings.

My first thought is that I must have been insane. I had just quit my old practice, exited the practice of medicine entirely, where I was on call for literally half the year! Why in heaven's name would I double that? Why throw myself into the deep end like that after I had just turned my back on the profession after a long period of burnout and unhappiness? It would seem to be a legitimate question – a question I would have been interested to ask anyone else who might have been in that situation. And yet, with the thought of creating something new, combined with my obvious insanity, in this place at the end of the planet, at the bottom of the earth, I did so without hesitation. It just seemed … *natural* for me to make the leap into that deep end. How strange.

My second thought, in retrospect, was how amazing it was that the nursing staff and radiographers would jump into that deep end with me, always willing to show up at any hour of the day or night. Whenever I would call, they would answer. The staff was not a large one and it required them to constantly shift their schedules around so that there would always be three nurses on call along with me, as well as a radiographer to run the x-ray equipment. This is the minimal number required to do a case in the cath lab. Not just my life was affected. Their lives, too, would also be forever interrupted at many an odd hour.

While our workplace was not a particularly large hospital, we would still get called in at least three times per week after hours (a number that would grow as the program matured). The staff would arrive within twenty minutes as soon as I activated the call back. In those early years, it was myself along with my incredibly committed and talented staff that made it all happen. To them I say, 'Thank you'.

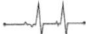

One Saturday afternoon, I found myself taking a walk through town to a location known as the Gorge. It is a place of natural beauty. A river runs through this section of town, fed upstream by a man-made lake, originally constructed for the production of hydroelectric energy. It was built in the late 1800s and became the first publicly owned hydroelectric power station in the Southern Hemisphere. Here, in the small town of Launceston. In the mid-20th century, additional construction was done to increase power generation, with the subsequent closure of the original turbines. The river, though, still flows through the section that housed those turbines and fills the 'basin', as it is called, a small lake-like body of water used for public swimming. Over this site sits a suspension bridge, originally built and opened in 1904. A large flood in 1929 caused destruction of the original bridge, but it was rebuilt and opened a few years later. It is a popular recreational area that has been developed over time, drawing both locals and tourists alike. I was new to the area, and so I had parked my car and walked the trail to arrive at the suspension bridge, taking in the surrounding woodlands, river, and wildlife.

It was then that my phone rang. A man in his forties was in the emergency room having a major heart attack resulting in cardiogenic shock. William was running a blood pressure of 70/30 with a pulse of 110 beats per minute. In the setting of a large heart attack, these are ominous numbers. And this is absolutely a time-sensitive case. I called the hospital operator to activate the call-back team.

Meanwhile, I found myself standing on the suspension bridge more than a kilometre away from my car, wearing, to my consternation, flip-flops. It would take at least twenty minutes to walk to my car. I was in no mood for a delay. I still had to get to Emergency, see the patient before he was moved, and, very typically in those early days, push the bed myself to the cath lab once I knew the nurses were there.

There was a time in my younger life when running felt as if I was floating on air. But that was in the past. I had given up running a few years earlier as I felt the havoc being perpetrated on my joints. Nevertheless, with my toes hanging on to those flip-flops, I took off and ran along the path to get out of the Gorge and get to my car. Probably one of the runs I remember more than any other (apart from one marathon twenty years earlier). Upon arrival at Emergency, I found myself with a man younger than I, with major ECG changes and a BP 70/40. William was ashen in colour and wearing an oxygen mask to help him breathe. The nurses had arrived, and the bed was pushed to the cath lab. It was not a simple fix, but we managed to finish the case and insert an intra-aortic balloon pump to help stabilize William's blood pressure. He was moved to the ICU, where the balloon pump would stay in for the next 72 hours. It was one of the first cases we had done in Launceston with a man this ill. He had survived getting through the angioplasty, and I gave him a fifty-fifty chance of survival at that point. Time is muscle.

Another day. Another call. It was 8 p.m. and I had just finished cleaning up after dinner. It was Emergency. A woman in her seventies was brought in with a very low blood pressure and chest pain for at least the preceding 24 hours. The history was now hard to obtain from her as she was quite ill and finding it difficult to answer questions. The ECG clearly showed that she was having a heart attack and again, the cath lab staff were called. On the table, the patient was in shock. Her right coronary artery was occluded with a normal left coronary system. Her BP was very low. I was not convinced that opening the artery would help. Much time had already passed since her symptoms began. The picture that she presented with bothered me. She 'looked' sicker than her anatomy. I performed a right heart catheterization to better understand the cardiac haemodynamics at play. On initial inspection, much like her coronary anatomy, the 'numbers' looked much better than she did. But then something dawned on me. One more measurement made the diagnosis. And this diagnosis was essential for the subsequent management decisions. Unfortunately, she had ruptured the septal wall that separates the right and left chambers of the heart. This was caused by her heart attack. But this does not happen acutely. It takes time, and always more than 24 hours. She chose not to come to hospital at the onset of symptoms when a coronary intervention might have saved her. She was presenting to us very late. Too late. There would be no angioplasty or open-heart surgery. The damage was irreversible. This type of intracardiac rupture is fatal. The case was stopped, and she passed away two hours later. Time is muscle.

Time. It is always playing out in the mind of an interventionalist. No more so than when one is on call.

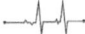

A man in his early seventies arrived at the Emergency triage desk having chest pain. He was standing there describing his pain to the triage nurse when he collapsed. He was then immediately put on a stretcher and taken to a resuscitation bed, where the Emergency staff went to work. CPR was commenced, as he had no spontaneous cardiac output or function. He was in ventricular fibrillation (VF) and was shocked with paddles. Briefly, so very briefly, he had a heart rhythm on the ECG with the clear diagnosis of an abrupt right coronary occlusion. He then went back into VF and CPR was re-commenced. This was the scenario when I arrived at the scene. This was very, very acute. It was happening right there. This occlusion had happened there in the Emergency Department and his heart rhythm, the electrical part of his heart, was trying to end his life. We had to get him to the cath lab.

This was the first case I would do with a Lucas device. The Lucas device is an electrically powered pneumatic pump that, once strapped onto the chest wall, will continue chest compression while the patient is being moved. A human is not required once the machine is on. The patient was brought into the lab with the Lucas doing CPR, as he had no effective heart rhythm. It is an imposing device, delivering external compressions far more powerful than any I had ever seen given by a human. Nevertheless, it is very effective, if a bit frightening to watch, given the power of its compressions. The patient was put on the table with this rather large apparatus strapped on his chest, and my job was to quickly visualize and fix the problem. I will just say that seeing around one of these devices is not simple. And the chest compressions that the Lucas device delivers are so strong that there is a lot of patient movement created while x-ray filming is underway. Performing an intervention under these circumstances is tricky. Maybe this was another day when I just got lucky. But I found the problem quickly and stented even quicker. With re-establishment of flow to this occluded vessel, we were then able to shock him back to normal and maintain both a normal rhythm and normal cardiac output. The Lucas device was removed as it was no longer required.

At the time of the coronary intervention, I had incidentally discovered that he also had critical disease in a second artery, but now was not the time to get distracted. The culprit vessel was fixed. We got him off the table. He woke up a few hours later.

Two days following this acute admission I brought him back to the lab and fixed the other critical problem. I subsequently saw him in my office a few months later. He remembered nothing. He had tried to die in front of us. It all happened so quickly. He was at the right place at a terrible time. Anywhere else, and he would never have survived. His heart had sustained no significant injury. He was back to normal. Time ...

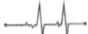

On call takes its toll. The night calls are the most difficult, as one would imagine. Waking at 2 a.m., going into the hospital, doing the work, going home, and then trying to get any sleep is its own skillset. It's common to return to bed only to be turning over the decisions you've made, the images of the anatomy flashing in your mind. When it goes smoothly and quickly, when it actually is 'straightforward', there is an opportunity to fall asleep. When the patient is ill, when the case is technically complicated, sleep is elusive.

There may be more than one call in a night. There is no rest the next day. Your schedule is fixed for the following day, whether you are back in the lab, or in the clinic, or in the office. When you are again on call that same day, the cycle can easily repeat itself. When you are on call 24/7, 365 days a year – I honestly do not know how I did that. And yet I did. And I loved it. Something must have been wrong with me.

It seems appropriate to call on yet another old adage, that what doesn't kill you makes you stronger. I don't know whether in this case that is true. I do know, however, that I became better, quicker, and smarter at what I do. In this business, there is no substitute for experience. And being on call for so many in those early days following my arrival, experience beyond my years of practice in the US was something coming fast and furious.

And William, that man with the 50/50 chance of survival? Twenty-plus years later, he is alive. Whenever I have seen him in the office since, I've always been greeted with a thank you and a hug from his wife. I have never forgotten the flipflops, the run, and the reasons, for all the hardships of being on call, why we do it.

CHAPTER 15
Galle

The only true voyage of discovery ... would be not to visit strange lands, but to possess other eyes, to see the universe with the eyes of another.

— Marcel Proust

In December 2004, a major tsunami struck off the coast of Indonesia, caused by an undersea earthquake. According to Wikipedia, it was the third most powerful earthquake recorded in history since modern seismographic measurements became available in the early 20th century. It would result in the deaths of nearly a quarter of a million people in at least 14 different countries in Asia. Sri Lanka was heavily hit with over thirty thousand deaths and the displacement of 1.5 million people. It resulted in a world-wide humanitarian relief effort with over US$14 billion donated from around the world.

Within a few years of the tsunami, I was to become involved in the relief effort. An Australian organization was created to help respond to the crisis in Sri Lanka. The Australian Sri Lankan Medical Assist Team (AUSLMAT) was started by a few Australian health professionals along with Sri Lankan expats living in Melbourne. They included general medical physicians and allied health care professionals, bringing much-needed medical equipment and medicine to Sri Lanka. The services provided would range from diabetes management to provision of eyeglasses or wheelchairs, anything that could be of use to a country recovering from a catastrophic natural disaster. One of the early organizers of the relief effort was a general cardiologist from Melbourne.

It is unlikely that I would have been drawn into this organization's relief efforts or would even have heard of it if not for Elizabeth. Of Anglo-Sri Lankan heritage, born and subsequently raised in a hill station in northern India within sight of the Himalayas, Elizabeth was one of the original cath lab nurses upon my arrival in Launceston, and would become my life partner. After the tsunami, her inherent connection to her heritage, along with her insistence on doing good things in the world, led her to contact AUSLMAT and offer our assistance. Thanks to the earlier efforts of Dr Jennifer Johns, the cardiologist involved in the beginnings of AUSLMAT, we were invited to help expand the interventional cardiac services being developed in the south of the country in the city of Galle.

Cardiac disease is rife in the developing nations of Southeast Asia and the subcontinent. With minimal governmental economic support provided at that time, we were asked to become involved. My initial visit was preceded by that of a colleague in Melbourne, Dr Omar Farouque, who was kind enough to give me a 'heads-up' on what to expect upon our arrival. He had found a staff very willing to learn and provide the necessary service. However, one disastrous case had occurred during his stay due to an inappropriately prepared medicine used in the cath lab, calling into question the safety of the drugs, and therefore all equipment available to us. It was his advice that we bring almost all the equipment and intracardiac medication we might need during the week we would be working there, and to check and reassess for ourselves the level of preparedness of this new lab. It was good advice, sorely worth heeding given the state of the service we found there.

Months before departing Tasmania for Sri Lanka, Elizabeth began coordinating the donation of equipment from a variety of cardiac device companies in Australia. We needed to provide most of the hardware we would be using, such as the balloons, guidewires, and stents. At the time, we really didn't know what to bring given that we had little to no idea of what we would find upon arrival. But it was fortunate that multiple device companies were kind enough to donate boxes of essential equipment, and we hoped it was enough to last the time we'd be there. Along with the equipment, given what had happened to the patient there the year before, specific medication used in intracardiac work was packaged and prepared for our trip.

While much of the general medical equipment that AUSLMAT sent to Sri Lanka was shipped via a cargo container, we were concerned that if the container did not arrive when we did (by no means guaranteed), then the whole trip would be a waste. Thus, we decided to pack the boxes and take them on the plane with us. Permission from the Sri Lankan Health Department had been given for the medical equipment to pass through Customs upon our arrival. Or so we were told.

On arriving in Colombo, we dutifully loaded our belongings onto the trolley, along with the boxes that had been packed with all our equipment, and headed out the baggage area door. Among the last to leave, we were stopped by an officer questioning us as to the content of said boxes. After we explained who we were, the aid organization we were with, and that we had been told that permission was given by the Health Minister for entry with the boxes, all were confiscated. We watched helplessly as our months of effort, bundled carefully in plastic wrap, complete with metallic wiring to encase the belongings, seemed to be rapidly disappearing. I need not say that this was very, very demoralizing. With little else to do, and having spent hours in the airport, we went to the group accommodation where the rest of the aid organization had gathered. We were fortunate that there were still a few days left before we were due at the hospital where we would be working, allowing for the head of our agency to contact the Health Ministry and arrange for the release of the medical equipment that had taken many months to secure.

We knew that there are no guarantees when it comes to timelines there, but as in almost all things, it's most often who you know that matters. And the Australian-Sri Lankan general physician running the show knew the Health Minister. A few phone calls were made and thus, within days, our boxes arrived at their destination, and in the nick of time as our planned first day was to begin.

We arrived at the hospital on the day and were escorted to the cath lab. It didn't take me very long to realize that I was somewhat of a curiosity. We were in a public hospital with over 2000 beds, the third-largest tertiary care centre in the country, providing care for millions of patients in the surrounding districts. There were people everywhere. Every corridor, every door frame, every bed, and often floor space next to the bed, was occupied by multitudes of people. There was laundry hanging off banisters and out of windows. Families providing cooked meals for their loved ones who'd been admitted into an available bed (or floor, as was often the case). And while I was walking through this morass of humanity, it was clear that I was the only Caucasian. It seemed as if everyone was staring at me. Not since high school had I found myself in the racial minority. I didn't know whether to feel embarrassed, bashful, important, or just plain self-conscious. It was interesting, to say the least.

After making our way through a myriad of corridors and stairwells, we arrived in the cath lab to find a brand new and quite pleasantly airconditioned room. Air conditioning was definitely not a common finding in this facility, but it was very, very welcome. The heat can be oppressive, and one could not help but note that large swathes of the outer walls of the hospital were typically covered in mould. But the lab was modern. And more importantly for everyone concerned, it was cool. Working with a lead apron on all day, along with the covering scrub gowns, significantly increases the temperature felt by those working in the room. I have worked without cooling systems in these environments. It does no one good to have sweat dripping into the eyes of the operator during a coronary intervention. Having air conditioning feels like a life saver.

I then met the cardiologist who was working there full-time, whom I was to work alongside. He was a pleasant guy with solid diagnostic skills, but only basic skills in coronary interventions. While the room was new, it contained no infrastructure other than the x-ray equipment. All the equipment we use on a routine basis merely sat on the floor. There were old boxes of gear lying there that had expiration dates from over six years earlier. How thankful we were that we had brought all the equipment that was donated to us. The nurses were not specifically trained at all in the cath lab, and their English was rudimentary at best. It was to be Elizabeth's job to train the nurses despite the clear language difficulties. She loved it. The challenges ahead were rife.

As with so many of my adventures in life, I arrived with no clear sense of what I was to do during the week I was to be there. I wished to help. I did not know if that meant I would stand and observe, proctor the cardiologist I met, or scrub as primary operator. All of the cases to be done had been pre-selected so that there would be no wasted time. They were then presented to me one at a time to be certain they were appropriate for intervention. A team of registrars and trainees were involved in getting patients to the hospital, as many of them had to travel long distances to get there.

I was quite overwhelmed and impressed by the degree of diligence and organization that was in place to maximize our time. Whatever may have been lacking in the lab, enthusiasm and preparedness with patients were not. I was yet to understand the skillset that was already there. There would effectively be no surgical backup for any complexities or complications that might arise, but having come from Launceston, I was quite used to that. During the week, the design and creation of a more effective, functional room was being attended to. Shelving needed to be purchased. Counters needed to be installed. Leaving boxes of unopened equipment lying on the floor simply would not do. But no time was to be wasted while all of this was taking place, and so the clinical work of seeing and fixing patients also began.

The first patient was a young man who had earlier been discovered to have critical disease in the right coronary artery. He was back for an elective PCI. I could not imagine what this must have been like for him. He did not speak English, and without the capacity to verbally engage with him, my age-old humour was not going to aid in making this easier for him. I had no idea if he knew what we were about to do, nor did I know what had been explained to him. He was only 37 years old. Besides the usual fears and apprehensions that any person has when undergoing coronary interventions, this was a very unusual procedure in this part of the world. And it just was not performed at this hospital. Did he feel a certain gratitude at having this done for him, at no monetary cost? Would having a man from Australia as the operator have created feelings of greater gratitude, or did it create even more fear? Was he thinking, *How rare is my problem, how difficult to fix if a man has to fly thousands of miles to come here and do this? Is that good or bad?* My speculations may all be absurd. For all I know, he was happy and excited to be there.

He was placed on the table, access was obtained by a junior doctor through the radial artery, and initial images were being obtained to start the case.

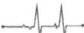

Meanwhile, I was struggling a bit. I was to discover that while I am not a particularly large man by any means, in Sri Lanka I seemed to be significantly above the average. I struggled to find scrub pants and a scrub shirt that would fit! I could barely get the shirt on over my head and shoulders. The pants, extending down to the top of my socks, were not a particularly good fashion statement. Next, I had to find a lead apron I could wear, and finally, a scrub gown before gloving.

In the western world, we have grown accustomed to one-use gowns that are disposed of. When I first started in Tasmania, we would use washable gowns, a practice that I assume ended based on the expense of maintaining a laundry service versus the cost of purchasing disposable ones. Fair enough. But I would find the laundered gowns in Galle not only quite short in the arms, but without elastic cuffs. Sterile gloves are meant to extend over the gown. To find the gown had no elastic at the wrist, with sleeves three times the diameter of your arms, kimono sleeves if you will, turned out to require a bit of arm-over-arm wrapping, while trying to secure the gloves around the sleeves, all while maintaining sterility.

While I am going through all of these frustrating gymnastics of finding a scrub top and getting my gloves on, I hear the consultant's voice ask me, 'Is it okay if the patient has ST elevations?' This is an ECG sign of a heart attack in progress. Not something an elective patient should have. So I first ask, 'Was it there when you started the case?' I'm thinking that perhaps this was a long-standing chronic ECG change. The answer is 'No'. Okay. That doesn't sound good. Well, what is happening here?

Finally able to get my gloves on, I move from the scrub sink through the room, which is now packed with people, including the cleaning staff, wanting to watch the events unfolding. I keep saying 'Excuse me', moving through a crush of staff in order to get to the head of the table, where lies a young man with major ECG changes on the monitor, a heart rate in the 30s and a BP of 70 systolic. I ask one of the nurses who can understand me if the patient is having any chest pain. She asks, now to find out his pain is being rated 10 out of 10. Next thing I see is that he is beginning to have dry heaves and retching. This is common when patients are having a heart attack. I ask to step into the primary operator position, with all the staff members moving steps to the right, because this is not good.

It is clear to me that the operator has inadvertently dissected the artery when he engaged or placed the catheter into the vessel, and there is now no blood flow. What disturbs me the most is that no one in the room recognizes what is happening, including the attending cardiologist who started the case. And no one knows what to do next. I've been there all of a few minutes, just trying to get my clothing on, and already we're having our first serious complication.

With all the equipment still in boxes on the floor, I now ask Elizabeth to find what I need to get things moving. Lots of running around the room ensues, searching for the devices we brought, and, fortunately, eventually, I am able to fix this young man without any further sequelae. His ECG normalizes, the pain subsides, and the vessel is successfully stented. He leaves the hospital later that day. My Sri Lankan colleague stands beside me at the end of the case, shaking his head back and forth. It's a good lesson for him to learn: how quickly things can go wrong. It happens to everyone. It's always about what you do next.

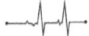

Over the course of the week, we would go on to do a couple of dozen cases. Often, I was in the room to merely guide my new-found colleague through the cases, offering advice on the next steps, what size stent to use, and so on. In most cases I needed to step in as the primary operator. Nevertheless, I saw my main role as a teacher. The purpose of us being there was to get a program up and running; to try to provide skillsets to both doctors and nurses so that after we left, they would be able to continue some of the work, even if not necessarily the most complex cases, in this very large public hospital servicing so many. Proverbially, we were teaching them how to fish … There are many levels of teaching, though, and not all are about technical skills.

I loved working with the nurses. They were all so keen to learn these skills. They were so shy. There was a large cultural difference obvious to us upon our arrival. In the western world, nurses work alongside physicians as coworkers, particularly in areas where technical skills are being used. No surgeon can operate without nursing assistance. No interventionalist can function without a skilled assistant alongside. In Sri Lanka, that kind of relationship did not exist. Doctors were perceived to be too many steps 'above' a nurse, both educationally and financially, so that the working relationship seemed to be more of co-existence rather than of colleagues.

Each day, there was a lunch break (a practice that I must say was new to me). The hospital would deliver cooked food to an adjacent room where we'd all go to have some nourishment and a chat about the work. On that first day, I remember sitting at a table with a plate of food in front of me alongside the other senior and junior doctors, the nurses standing at the entrance door. Just standing there. They were waiting for us to finish eating before they would enter. Eating with and alongside the doctors was a behaviour that was not commonly done by the nurses. But this would not do. Certainly not for Elizabeth. She immediately shepherded them into that room, encouraging them to be a part of the team. They would not be 'less than'. I loved that. I really did.

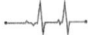

There was one nurse I took a particular liking to. Perhaps because of her eagerness. Or her shyness, and her kind smile. She did not speak English. When she scrubbed at the table with me, I would encourage her to do some simple, but important physical task. Each time she would go to do what I had asked of her, I would lean to my right and bump her hands. She would look at me as if she had done something wrong. I would nod my head and tell her to go ahead. As she'd start, again the bump … Again, the look. Once again, 'Please go ahead'. A third time, the bump, her look at me, followed by my smile and laugh. Then she understood: it was a joke. The best I could do in the realm of slapstick humour with someone who could not speak with me. I would end up doing a version of that over a number of years with new nurses in Launceston, but it started in Galle.

We ended up completing a couple of dozen interventional cases that week. Some were tough. I was able to proctor my colleague through many of them and was confident he had learned a great deal. I hoped everyone had learned a great deal, including the cleaning staff so eager to watch! By the end of the week, we had nearly run out of equipment. I had to factor in, for each case, what was to be used and what was left over, hopeful that some critical device was available when we needed it. The calculations worked out pretty well in the end.

The room evolved into a functional cath lab by the time the shelving and counters were put in and all the boxes were emptied. I considered this to be a very successful and fruitful experience for everyone involved. When we left to return home, we were given parting gifts from the staff. It had been a great privilege and honour to be entrusted with this responsibility of teaching and working with staff so far from home. The best gifts, however, were their warmth and kindness. And the food! The food was fantastic!

I think the nurses really loved Elizabeth. She was their

champion. They cried that final day. When it was time for us to go, I made a speech directed to the nurses on how important their role was in that room. That doctors could not do everything by themselves; they needed and depended on each and every one of the nurses to help them, to help the patient. They would be silent no longer. You could almost feel their sense of empowerment grow. I think after that day they stood a little taller. It was all part of the mentoring of this unique experience.

Teaching: it has so many forms.

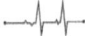

We returned two years later to proctor and teach once again. Much had changed in that time. Sri Lankan doctors now would leave the island, train elsewhere, and return to their homeland, bringing new and advanced skills to the country. When I arrived this second time, I thought that maybe my experience and skill were no longer required. The lab had progressed, and coronary interventions were routinely being done. The nursing staff were far more experienced and assertive in their role. It was gratifying to have played some part in that progression. I discovered that perhaps I still had a thing or two to teach them. My role as primary operator remained for a number of difficult cases, but it was clear to me that it would only be a matter of time before guys like me were no longer necessary. It was another reminder that for any of us, our time on centre stage is limited. We learn, we do, we teach ... and the world moves on.

Going to Galle was a much smaller investment of time, but like Launceston, it provided a chance for me to help create something new. I loved it. And I am forever grateful for the opportunity.

CHAPTER 16
Complications

I am a great believer in luck. The harder I work, the more I seem to have.

— Coleman Cox

After literally tens of thousands of angiograms, and thousands of coronary interventions, you might imagine and even expect there are many stories to tell. There really are. But they're not stories in those moments. When you stand at the table with the patient lying in front of you, you are snapped into the reality that no matter what it looks like on the x-ray screen, this ain't no video game. And when things do not go well, when the procedure is not rolling on smoothly according to the master plan, life just gets a little bit harder. And so you accumulate an experience over years of time. I feel as if I have seen it all. Witnessed the worst outcomes, and the greatest saves. The cases mount in your mind. You get smarter, more efficient, learn to avoid the pitfalls, hopefully dodge the bullets. And yet no matter how experienced, how 'good' you are, things keep on happening. Those 'happenings' being what you are not expecting.

You have read enough to know that whatever it is that you are not expecting, is something you could happily do without. How else can I express this feeling? I will say it again. This is a crazy way to live, and a crazy way to make a living.

So many events over so many years. The volume of cases that I was to perform in Tasmania placed me as one of the busiest operators in the country. It has made some of my stories harder to remember as the volume grew: I suppose that it's only natural, to fail to remember when the numbers, the faces, the anatomy become so many. Some just stay with you, lingering in the back of your thoughts, your memories. Those that have stayed with me, as you might imagine, are those that have had the most impact on both my life and the lives of others. That impact may be either good or bad. And each, whether good or bad, has its own set of repercussions and consequences. This emotional toll that the work can take is felt by all in the room. The nurses and radiographers carry the wins and the losses in their own way, even if different from my own.

The consequences of this work may last a day, a week, or a lifetime (as I tell many of these stories decades after the fact). One thing is certain: in the midst of the battle, on the day that I stand at that table, I only see me and the patient. For me, nothing else is important. This may turn into war, a war between the disease I see, and what I have to do to win the fight. Sometimes it's slam dunk straightforward, other times a fight for survival. I am a guy in the trenches, alongside the patient. This is personal.

—⋀⋀—

Bill was an 80-year-old man admitted with a worrisome cardiac history of breathlessness and chest pain. I had met him the day before taking him to the cath lab. While Bill was still living at home, with some assistance from his daughter, I did not think that he was a good candidate for open heart surgery, should that have been part of the treatment options to consider. Well before any cardiac procedure is to start, we begin the process of risk assessment. This risk assessment can often be complicated, and is dependent on many variables including age, kidney function, heart muscle function, cognitive impairment, other chronic illnesses (co-morbidities), and the overall cardiac anatomy, to name a few. Each case takes these multiple variables into account before a final treatment decision is made. The options also include medication alone. Not everything needs to be mechanically 'fixed'. Assessing Bill, I had already concluded that his risks for open heart surgery were very high and this would not be a viable option, even as the case began.

Bill was on the table for a diagnostic study where it was discovered that he had a worrisome, critically narrowed left circumflex coronary just at its origin (ostium). This was considered an extremely risky PCI given the location and the size of the artery. It was a huge vessel, compensating for a rather tiny right coronary artery. Having already concluded that he was a poor surgical candidate, we gave Bill intravenous heparin (blood thinner), and I began the work of stenting this high-grade, tight lesion. Following one balloon dilatation, all hell broke loose. He arrested on the table and a code blue was called.

The ICU team quickly arrived, and Bill was intubated and placed on a ventilator. While he was being 'tubed', that is having a breathing tube placed through the mouth, it was clear from a subsequent image that he had formed an occlusive thrombus (clot) in the left main artery, adjacent to where the balloon was inflated. This thrombus extended into the origins of both major vessels, the circumflex and left anterior descending. There was minimum flow anywhere. Yet another example of the speed at which these events are witnessed in this subspecialty: from stable to critical with inflation of a tiny balloon.

At that time, we had a new instrument in the lab able to measure or quantify the amount of blood thinner the patient had received. While this is now a routine measurement done in virtually all labs around the world, there was a time when this was not the case. But having it then was essential for what transpired. A blood sample was quickly drawn up, demonstrating that Bill's anticoagulation was profoundly too low, that is, his blood was not thin enough. Despite the fairly hefty dose I had given him at the beginning of the procedure, the drug had 'tissued,' meaning it never got into his circulation. The IV cannula was not positioned in the vein properly and the blood thinner had been delivered into subcutaneous tissue. Without the blood thinner on board, his blood quickly formed a clot at the site where the balloon was inflated. And this clot was in a location very, very hazardous to his survival. Much like the business of real estate sales, the risk of arterial blockages is often about location, location, location – Bill was nearly gone in the blink of an eye.

After giving him another blood thinner dose directly into his coronary vessel, I started the work of clot removal and re-establishing flow in both affected arteries. His other leg was prepped and I quickly inserted an intra-aortic balloon pump to help with the minimal coronary flow still present.

In these moments when so much is happening at the table, it is as if three things need to be done simultaneously. The battle in the trenches has become serious. Prioritizing what is to be done first, having the technical skills to perform quickly, and most importantly, communicating with the team around you, become vital to the outcome. There was much to do. Yet with all that was happening, what most struck me about the case, what I remembered the most, was when the ICU doctor who had responded to the code, looked at me and suggested that I stop. Stop doing anything. As we say in the business, call it. His estimation was that the likelihood of survival was poor, and that continuing on was fruitless, and perhaps even cruel. I admit that the thought crossed my mind, ever so briefly. But only briefly. This man came in the door talking, and something happened to him on the table. All because an IV cannula was not working properly! That doesn't seem like a good reason to die! When they're talking to you as they come into the room, they are supposed to be talking on the way out.

Despite this not being a quick and easy fix, we got him through the case. He survived. Barely. After adequate blood thinners were delivered, and a few stents later, he was sent to ICU with a reasonable blood pressure, and a balloon pump operating while he remained on a ventilator. He would stay in hospital for the next week or so and fully recover. Weeks later, I received a photo of Bill, taken by his grateful daughter, sitting on the farm surrounded by his farm animals.

This story is one that is not easily forgotten. Yes, I was emotionally gratified, as was the patient and family. And yes, I was equally gratified to have the technical skills to complete the work. To do battle. Yet there was a third factor at play here that was of great importance to me, as it weighed on my mind during the events unfolding. Another lesson long ago learned.

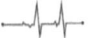

Despite my 'seniority' as an operator, I like to think that I have always been willing and able to listen to what others say. Take into account the opinions of others in a specialty where the answer is not black and white, where the 'grey zone' is forever present. I have worked alongside some smart and talented operators over the years. And have learned a vast number of techniques as the specialty evolved. But always, without a doubt, when it comes to having to 'make the call', the big choice, in the heat of the battle, I listen to myself first. This is not an easy thing to be said. And I mean that sincerely. It may even sound a bit condescending to many of my colleagues. A senior ICU doctor is telling me to let it go. Stop … the likelihood of survival is poor. This belief in listening to self is not a given. It has to grow and be nurtured with that thing called experience. This does not happen overnight. We are all full of self-doubts. It is the nature of the human condition. I have done plenty of second guessing along the way. It is not about being without doubts, it's what you do next that matters.

It began with a very specific case so many decades ago, when I did not have the experience, nor the confidence, to make the final decision. There were other opinions. Other voices that made it all sound so clear. I let it happen. I was relatively junior, so I tell myself. And he paid the price.

In the middle of a PCI, before the advent of stents, the angioplasty failed, resulting in the sudden complete occlusion of an artery. Despite this sudden anatomic change, the patient, a man in his fifties, remained pain free with no obvious changes on the ECG. When the cath lab staff saw the vessel was lost, the surgical suite was immediately notified, and before I knew it the chief surgeon was up in the cath lab looking at the films. I had not even called him. It was a quick reflex by staff in an era when such complications were not uncommon. As I was pondering the situation, thinking of what to do, or even if anything should be done given the patient's stability, the operating theatre was being prepared. Phone calls were being made, and a trolley was being pushed into the lab to take the patient for emergency surgery. Meanwhile, he remained pain free, and I was still asking myself, *why are we going to do surgery when he is fine?* A final angiographic image revealed that the occluded vessel was receiving collateral flow from another artery, explaining the absence of ECG changes and clinical stability. Again, I was asking myself, *do we need to operate on this patient?* But the tide was against me at that moment with so many moving parts already in motion. What if I didn't send him for surgery and something happened later? How could I know? What were the long-term consequences of leaving him as he was with an occluded vessel? I just caused this – didn't we have to fix it? Or did we? Everyone else seemed to think that doing surgery was the right thing to do! Who was I to think differently? So, despite my reservations, I allowed the patient to be wheeled out for emergency surgery. Who was I …?

The next day, following his operation, I went to see him in ICU, only to discover that he was now critically ill. He had developed multiorgan failure including kidney, cardiac, and liver. All likely due to the bypass operation. He was in a coma that would last for weeks, on renal dialysis for weeks. Further complications were to set in later. His 'recovery' was catastrophic. Ultimately, he failed to leave the hospital. All of this from a 'low-risk' single vessel bypass surgery in a low-risk individual. I had told myself all this when they wheeled him away. I thought it was low risk. I had relented to the opinion of others. Again, who was I … I would not be so easily persuaded again. If this occurred today, there is no way I would allow him to go to surgery. There is no need. His prognosis would be fine. We know a lot more after three decades. These are the outcomes that haunt you forever.

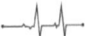

Another tale. A different story.

I was doing a procedure called rotational atherectomy. What I am about to relate may sound a bit crazy. Having been around when it first became available decades ago, I too, thought it insane. We use a diamond-tipped high speed 'drill' or burr to create a path in an artery that is heavily calcified. Yes, we drill the inside of the artery, and it takes a diamond-tipped drill. When calcific plaque causes obstruction to blood flow, it can be difficult to open with stents. It is akin to trying to prise two large boulders apart with a balloon inserted in a crack between the two. The balloon is likely to burst before the boulders move a millimetre. And so it is with heavily calcified arteries. Opening such a hard blockage with a balloon risks balloon rupture and possible perforation of the vessel. The only way to open such physically hard vessels is to literally soften them a bit. We often choose to approach this problem by drilling through the calcium with what effectively is a drill bit rotating between 150,000–200,000 rpm. It sounds much like a dentist's drill. Once the artery is remodelled by the drill bit, the process is followed up with stent deployment. This sounds a little nuts, and quite dangerous, but it is a very effective tool in the right circumstances. And when it works smoothly.

During this specific 'procedure', the burr or drill bit moved quickly through the calcified section. Too quickly. And I now could not remove it! The diamond-tip drill only has the diamonds on the front end for crossing the blockage. The back side is smooth. The burr passed through the calcified area, but much like an old Chinese finger trap; once in, I could not get it out! I was pulling and pulling, but it was absolutely stuck inside the patient's artery. It is important to state that this is (fortunately) not a common complication, but unfortunately for me, it was not one I had ever seen before.

So here, yet again, I was to find myself with a problem – a problem created by me – that I had not encountered before. It was not the first time that some creative thinking alongside preparation would come in handy. How can I convey what it's like to be standing at the table with a diamond-tipped drill bit stuck inside the patient's heart? And they're awake!

Part of building the teaching program from the bottom up was to be prepared for anything that I could imagine – and even what I could not. I had spent a considerable amount of thinking time contemplating all the things that could go wrong in the cath lab. (By now, I suspect you have come to see how many things can happen.) It was equally important to acquire the necessary equipment to have on hand to deal with those complications (preparedness). I also needed to know and/or learn how to use those pieces of equipment that were not part of the day-to-day but were essential in an emergency. This time, it seemed like fate intervened. I had recently read an article published from a UK hospital of a technique that someone had described in a very similar situation, when the burr, or drill bit, was stuck in an artery. So, I decided, one more time, to do something I had never seen or done.

It is difficult to describe on paper, even to someone familiar with the equipment. Having never seen it done, it was not so different for me. In this one confusing sentence I am about to write, I cut the burr and its cable from its housing, slid a smaller catheter over the wire hanging out of the patient, and pushed it forcefully in, managing to capture the burr inside the new catheter I had inserted. With that, I removed everything together and voila, the burr was out. (Do not be concerned if this doesn't makes sense. It is just another set of crazy, once in a lifetime manoeuvres.) This very slick technique, once begun, had taken me all of 60 seconds, just one minute to bail myself out of a rather sticky problem. A thought experiment, one that I had read and rehearsed in my mind, put into action! And with success! Moments like this make you want to turn to the audience and to take your bow to thunderous applause! Not every day do you see this done. In the nearly twenty years since, I have not seen this happen again. But this was not the time to take my bow. I had managed to correct a big mistake, but the case was far from finished. I reinserted another, larger burr to make the opening in the calcified artery bigger, then finished the stent deployment. Later that same day the patient was home enjoying a glass of wine on his deck. I walked away with another sense of dodging the bullet. Another story remembered. Another lesson learned.

Then there was the time that a similar diamond-tipped rotational burr cut right through the wall of the artery. Punched a hole clean through. This is the most feared and dreaded complication of using a high-speed drill bit inside an artery. You must fix this, and quickly, to avoid a mortality on the table. With some effort, a stent covered with polyurethane (a so-called covered stent) was inserted, sealing off the leak. For years we had these covered stents on the shelf, rarely ever used. But when you need it, you are eternally thankful you have it. The lesson reinforced: think, prepare, always learn.

So many stories. So many battles in the trenches.

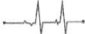

While trying to insert a stent to the appropriate location through a resistant segment of yet another artery in yet another patient, I lost the stent in the anterior descending artery. It came off the balloon before the balloon had been expanded. Stents are 'crimped' onto the balloon in the factory with significant force. They do not readily come off the balloon when moving them through the circulation. However, if pushed and pulled enough in tissue that is diseased with plaque, the stent can be stripped off the balloon. And so you are left with this tiny piece of metal sort of 'floating' around in the coronary circulation until it lodges itself somewhere. This was far from the first time this had happened to me, I might add. In this particular case, I managed to spear the unopened stent with another balloon catheter and pull it out. It is pretty hard to do that. Never seen it done before, nor since. I had a deep sense of satisfaction. My radiographer still has the photo we took of that 'speared' and recovered stent. But no bow – the case isn't done. More equipment is taken out of its packaging, I continue, and eventually the case is completed.

I have lost stents in other arteries as well. Part of the problem in retrieving a lost stent is that they are not easily visualized with the x-ray equipment. When they are not yet open or expanded, and come off the deployment balloon, the profile is so small that they can be near impossible to see, let alone to fish out. And recall that the thickness of the stent is on average 80 microns! I have had occasions where the optimal choice is to just crush the stent to the side of the vessel and put another stent in, covering the crushed one. Yeah, stent the stent.

One day, the stent came off the delivery balloon while in the aorta, outside the coronary tree. I watched as this tiny piece of metal spun around, yes, spun around like a top, and then disappeared. Gone off the screen! I had no idea where it went. Internally, I admit that I was a bit freaked out. If it went to the brain, we were all in big trouble – most of all the patient. I asked him how he was. He was fine. I took the x-ray equipment and scanned his head and his abdomen. No sign of the stent. Again, nearly impossible to see. After waiting a few minutes, with no clinical sign of a problem, I proceeded and fixed the problem we were there to fix. I saw him months later. He had no sign of anything untoward happening. Wherever it ended up in his circulation, was obviously not of clinical concern. Sometimes, it's just luck that gets you through.

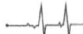

I wish it was only the heart that one had to worry about.

The problem, the complication, is not always with the heart. It can occur in other parts of the circulation. I was trying to get a catheter in the femoral artery, found around the crease where the leg meets the abdomen, in an elderly gentleman with severe stenosis (narrowing) of the aortic valve. It was a difficult access. It was hard to feel his pulse adequately and thus where to aim the insertion needle. I ultimately hit the artery with a needle but could not thread a wire or catheter into the vessel. The man now began to bleed heavily, and I was pushing hard on his groin to control the haemorrhage. His blood pressure was falling, and I knew time was limited. Patients with aortic stenosis do not tolerate blood loss well and when their BP is dropping, this is an ominous sign. While receiving help with compression from one of the nurses, I gained access to the femoral artery in the patient's left leg. After I inserted a catheter into his lower abdomen, a picture confirmed where he was bleeding from.

Switching gear, we were able to deploy a covered coronary stent into the artery that was bleeding and stop the haemorrhage. Once things were under control, I finished the diagnostic study, and he would be sent for an elective valve replacement. While this procedure on a more peripheral blood vessel was not standard teaching during my training, working with little surgical backup had taught me to do many things I would not have otherwise done.

Another non-cardiac problem. While trying to gain access to the femoral vein (which sits adjacent to the femoral artery) in a patient for a procedure to close a congenital hole in the heart, another mishap, so to speak, occurred. Gaining access to a femoral vein is rarely accompanied by complications. It is a low-pressure environment with minimal acute bleeding problems. So it was much to my surprise that, following a difficult access and finally the closing of this intracardiac hole, the patient was not looking good and was lethargic with low blood pressure. An emergency CT scan showed retroperitoneal blood, a bleeding problem that could only be caused by the puncture of some vascular structure that I was not aiming for. Again, I had never seen this happen with venous access. Never. And I had done thousands.

Once the bleeding was confirmed, we had to put the patient back on the table and access the left femoral artery to get appropriate imaging. Lo and behold, the first image showed a fistula between the femoral vein and a small branch of another artery (called the inferior epigastric artery). A fistula is an abnormal connection bridging two structures not normally communicating with one another. In this case, the two structures were a vein and a very small branch of an artery that have nothing to do with each other. The needle puncture had inadvertently passed through both vessels, and after the gear was removed from the patient, the abnormal connection remained, as she was bleeding internally. Badly.

Having by now learned many new techniques with different equipment, I was able to manipulate a very small delivery catheter into this tiny, bleeding artery that had formed a fistula, and deploy a small coil (a device previously seen used to clot off a coronary perforation) causing it to immediately clot off. The effect was immediate. The loss of this small vessel was of no damaging consequence. The internal bleeding was stopped and the blood that was there would be broken down by the body and reabsorbed into the surrounding tissue. Following an overnight stay, the patient would walk out of the hospital. Another bullet dodged.

Dodging the bullet. That is, sort of, what it feels like in those moments. A childhood dream of superhero moves, the guy who saves the day, becoming reality. Yet I know that the bullet is headed for the patient, not me, and I am the one who shot the bullet to start with. I create the problem. I have to fix it. In those moments of fear, stress, and generalized anxiety, it *feels* as if the bullet is coming for me. It is as if I have to save the patient, and in the process, save myself. You might begin to see why I think of this a bit as trench warfare.

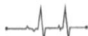

Reading these stories, these cases that have shaped who I have become as a cardiologist as well as a human being, can be overwhelming. Many of the details, particularly the anatomy, may not be fully understood by the reader. The totality of reading one after another, even for an experienced operator, is a bit over the top! I dare say it would be a challenge for any physician who does not work in these anatomic areas to follow the details of what I have written. I apologize for the volume. Yet all of this is important in gaining an appreciation of what can be harrowing complexity. And remember, I am describing a lengthy list of complications that *may* occur. These are the cases that guys like me go over in their minds, often for years. The reader should not think that this is common. Ninety-nine per cent of the time, diagnostic and interventional cases have no complications whatsoever. Given the good outcomes of this kind of work, and the thoughtfulness that interventionalists employ in decision making, I would truly hope that reading these stories would *never, never* dissuade the reader from taking appropriate advice from their cardiologist. But this is the life I have had. These are the stories that have stayed with me, the complex problems encountered over decades.

I like to believe that I have become a reasonable operator over the years. Much of my skill has come from experiences like these – problems arising that I had never seen, with no backup to help. And, important to note, problems that I have created myself! Patients may be stable, may be ill, may even be critical, but these kinds of complications are created by the interventionalist. No one shows up in the room with any of this. I have no intent to frighten the reader with these stories, but while the techniques have become more refined over time, and we often make the majority of the work we do look easy, it is not.

You can see that after decades, the stories of complications can make up a long and significant list. Each has lessons to teach; each provides something to learn. The ones I remember are, again, those with the greatest impact. In the telling, I hope the reader gains some insight into this little-written-of subspecialty where successes far outweigh the failures, yet should never, ever, be taken for granted. This small fact is of particular importance. The success rate of all coronary interventions routinely exceeds 96 per cent. The 'failures' are usually cases where the outcome is not what was hoped for, but no damage was done. It is less than 1 per cent of all patients who are placed on the table who may run into real trouble. It is in those precarious moments when it makes a difference that the operator, standing at the head of the table, knows what to do next. Over the extent of my career, I have come to see this as a game of millimetres. When the blood vessels we work inside of range in size from 2 to 7 millimetres, it doesn't take much for things to go from stable to critical, again, in the blink of an eye. So you think ahead, prepare for whatever may happen, and keep learning.

I have mentioned a few times in the span of my career that some days you are better off being lucky than good. But I agree with Coleman Cox on this point. The harder you work, the luckier you will become.

CHAPTER 17
Home stretch

Two roads diverged in a wood, and I—
I took the one less travelled by,
And that has made all the difference.

—Robert Frost

It remains vivid in my memory, driving south on the Major Deegan (a highway named for an early 20th-century political leader and major in the Army Corps of Engineers) with my father at the wheel, once again accompanying him to his work. I was about ten years old. To my right, parallel for a distance, the Hudson River. Spanning the Hudson further south was the George Washington Bridge, which leads to New Jersey. For me, the Hudson River was big. And New Jersey was another world away from the Bronx. There was a 1970s cover of *The New Yorker* I had seen in my teens, depicting a portion of Manhattan occupying 70 per cent of the frame, stretching from 9th Avenue westward to the Hudson, with New Jersey as a sliver. This was then followed by the continental US, the Pacific Ocean, and far in the distance, seen as little islands, Japan, China, and Russia. Seventy per cent of the frame, a portion of NYC, thirty per cent the rest of the world. This was how New Yorkers viewed the planet. As if from the centre. Everything else occupying little space. Who would have dreamed that I would one day be in Tasmania?

My father had wanted me to be a dentist. A practical man whose main concerns were making a living, improving his golf game, and having his children obtain a better life, he saw dentistry as a solid profession, good money, and no calls at night. My mother reached further, wanting me to be an orthodontist. She clearly saw Americans clamouring for their children to have beautiful smiles! While in high school, I asked my father how much longer I would have to be in school to become a dentist. He told me that it would take four years of university education followed by four years of dental school. If you have absorbed any of what I had written in the chapter touching on my earlier life, you will know that my aversion to school was real and it was immutable. And there was no way in hell I was going to go to school for eight more years after I finished high school! Who would have imagined that I would spend *twenty* more years in education and training before I would be gainfully employed?

During my second year of high school, there was a prolonged teachers' strike in New York City from the beginning of September, ending only in November. I was thrilled. Parents were not impressed. The following year another strike was looming before the start of the school year and my parents were apprehensive about my ongoing education, even if I was not concerned in the least. I was a product of the public school system of the Bronx. Yet my father came to me just prior to the (potential) start of grade 11 and asked if I would like to attend a private school in Manhattan. I knew of no one who went to a private school. This was not something seen in my neighbourhood. It was something I had never even considered, but with the teachers' strike a possibility, and having viewed their impressive brochure (yes, I thought it looked very cool) I thought I might have a look. We subsequently drove to the school, in the middle of the city, to visit, and I began to see the potential advantages of private education. The school was small, although everything was small compared to my school. It was attended by girls as well as boys. Clearly, this would have been a very significant change for me. Most importantly, as someone who had been 'schooled' and trained in the streets and schoolyards of New York, I was infinitely confident I could play on any sports team that they had. So there were pros: smaller size, sports stuff ... and girls.

Then there was the cons. I had to leave the few friends I had begun high school with. I would have to travel on the subway every day to school. I would have to wear a school uniform with a tie and blazer! What? In those days we were already wearing jeans to school, a very novel change to the standard attire that had existed for generations. A tie and blazer seemed a bit over the top. I wasn't totally dissuaded by having to take the train, but at the end of the day, the blazer was not for me, and I liked the guys I was hanging out with at school. Such are the life decisions made by a 14-year-old. I never went to private school.

It is not lost upon me how life might have been altered had a few choices been made differently. I suspect that many of us who might have reason to reflect on the past have gone through this ultimately useless exercise. Nevertheless, one thing does lead to another. If I had taken that path to private school, *maybe* the dominoes would have fallen in another direction. Maybe Ivy League university, followed by prestigious institutions, important friends with connections, wealthy women …! Hahahaha. The imagination can run wild, and rarely in a bad direction, always looking to what's greener, as they say.

Yet all those other singular moments that changed the course of my story would never have happened, starting with one chat with my sister. That one dog. One friend. One application accepted. Alter the path and none of it happens. The successes I would ultimately find in my life were certainly delayed, to say the least. The early years of practice were to be a mere warm up, and a huge learning experience, for what would come later. I don't know whether this following sentiment is just to make me feel better about my life, but I really do think there is much to be said for success that follows difficult times, and yes, even failure. Maybe early success is a trap. I don't know. I never had it. It just strikes me that later success maybe, just maybe, feels a bit sweeter, a tad more satisfying, and very, very gratifying. You can't look up until you've been down, you can't understand warmth unless you've been cold, and you can't taste the sweetness unless you have known the sour. I can only say that my own personal and professional resurrection was deeply, deeply satisfying.

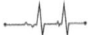

A few years ago, I was yet again called in from home to help an associate who was 'stuck'. No interventionalist likes to call for help when they feel they are capable of completing a case on their own. But this was already an after-hours call back, and he had been at the table for nearly an hour struggling to start what I would call the first step of the intervention. The tiny guidewire used to pass the balloons and stents inside the artery is first passed through the blockage. After all of this time had transpired, this first step was still not completed. It can be a very difficult step, or very easy. It is often the point of no return. Once done, it's up to the operator to finish the case.

In any event, I was asked to come in and assist. I arrived, changed, scrubbed for the case, and taking over as primary operator, passed the wire, literally in ten seconds. Less than ten minutes later, the case was completed, and the grateful cath lab staff could pack up and go home. I know that sometimes luck has played a role in a successful outcome, but more often it is skill.

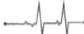

This story reminds me of a tale about Pablo Picasso. There are numerous versions, and its authenticity is questionable. While sitting at a restaurant, he was approached by a diner who was a great fan, who then asked Picasso if he could make a sketch for him. Picasso agreed, and after ten minutes using a pencil and a napkin, he produced a picture. He then told the diner that it would cost $100,000. The diner, who was shocked, said, 'But it only took you ten minutes! How can you possibly charge so much money?!' To which Picasso replied, 'It is not ten minutes. It is forty years and ten minutes.'

This last emergency case was not the ten minutes it took me to complete. It has taken me over three decades to be able to do cases in this time. It is a bit oxymoronic to say, but it takes a long time to do something, in a short time! And this was not a solitary event by any means. One of our beginner nurses once asked the senior nurses why I seemed to get the easiest cases, judging ease by time taken. When I heard the comment, I could only laugh.

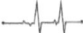

Interventional cardiology has come a very, very long way in the time I have been involved. While the subspeciality has its origins and core in coronary work, it has dramatically expanded. Devices are now routinely deployed to correct any one of a variety of other non-coronary problems. We fix congenital 'holes' linking chambers that should be separated by a wall. Devices are placed into small appendages in the heart to prevent blood clots forming. Aortic stenosis, the most common acquired valvular problem of aging, is now routinely fixed using percutaneous (through a small puncture in the skin) techniques rather than open heart surgery. Problems with other valves such as the mitral and tricuspid valves, not covered in this text, are more and more becoming a target of the interventionalist. Electrophysiology, an entire additional subspeciality of cardiology dealing exclusively with electrical matters of the heart, was created with the development of interventional tools and procedures. Nevertheless, despite all of this growth, the centre of it all remains in coronary work. In Table 1 I have compiled a simplified list of the 'tools' available when I began versus the tools of today. If nothing else, it is an indicator of the progress made.

Table 1: Development of tools and procedures in Interventional Cardiology

	1985	**2024**
Equipment	Balloon	Balloon
	Guidewire	Guidewire
	Intra-aortic balloon pump	Intra-aortic balloon pump
		Stents (dozens of designs)
		Covered stents
		Intravascular ultrasound
		Rotational atherectomy
		Intravascular lithotripsy
		Vascular coils
		Coronary doppler flow wires
		Coronary pressure wires
		Trapping balloons
		Guiding catheter extensions
		Optical coherence tomography
		Microcatheters
		Guide catheter extenders
Blood Thinning Drugs	Heparin	Heparin
	Aspirin	Enoxaparin (low molecular weight heparin)
		Thrombolytics (to dissolve clots)
		Aspirin
		Clopidigrel
		Ticagrelor
		Tirofiban
Intracoronary Drugs		Verapamil
		Adenosine
		Nitroglycerine
		Acetylcholine

In addition to these tools, the catheters have reduced in size by 33–50 per cent and advances in materials technology have made the delivery of balloons and stents somewhat easier (although, again, I use with caution the word 'easy'). The list also minimizes the sheer number and types of balloons and stents now available, along with the engineering of the guidewires used. These wires alone can make or break a case.

Many, many techniques for delivery of stents have evolved in this time, far beyond the purview of these writings. I remember listening to an excellent lecture on the complex subject of opening up chronically blocked coronary arteries, those vessels totally obstructed for months to years. Even in this subspecialty, the techniques the speaker was describing have been mastered by few. He went on to outline the nine different technical skillsets you needed to possess to be a successful operator in this very specific arena. At the time, I was happy that I had at least six or seven of these skills. The average operator has three or four. Having those three or four techniques is enough to perform over 90 per cent of cases. But when things get complicated …

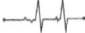

Not so many weeks ago, I was 'intervening' on a tightly narrowed bifurcation case of the right coronary. Very tightly narrowed. Ms Johnson had presented with fairly typical angina getting worse by the day. Her other vessels were normal. The decision to move forward with PCI was an obvious one.

Step one, as I have noted above, is passing one of the small guidewires through the initial narrowing. I had already used three different wires with no success. So, step one was yet to be completed. This was not easy. As I was manipulating the fourth wire chosen (each wire with different physical characteristics), a slight stain of contrast was noted at the point of narrowing. This was a sign that a small dissection was forming. At this juncture I was getting a bit concerned. Bail out now, stop the proceedings before things really, really go bad, or go for it? There was no room for mistakes now. Fortunately, with the fourth wire, I managed to get through the narrowing, followed by a serious sigh of relief on my part. But this was, to repeat, only step one.

The rest of the case did not go smoothly. I struggled each and every step, until two hours later, the stents were deployed. I let Ms Johnson know everything looked great as I also related that this was not a typical case. I didn't want her to think it always took so long. Internally, I had felt that bullet whizzing past once again. But that feeling doesn't just go away.

Months have passed since. I close my eyes and still see the arteries. I still see the wires. I still feel the struggle of passing the wires and balloons and stents through this diseased vessel. I see the finished images. These tough cases simply don't just go away after you are finished. This is not a unique 'aftershock'. And it is not a part of the work I have ever enjoyed.

Every time I have been involved in difficult cases and complex interventions, the images are seared into my brain. I see them when I go to sleep at night. In the midst of a normal conversation with someone, while words are being exchanged, I see wires moving along the vessel pathway. I see and feel the resistance to the push of the equipment, the calcification of the vessel wall. Should I have done this, or should I have done that? All of this taking place in my thoughts during an unrelated conversation, hidden from anyone but me. It is a disturbing, and unwelcome ongoing distraction. After the case is done, I relive the moments, the anatomy imprinted on my retina. Before an impending complex case, I mentally practice the moves, the techniques, prepare for what to do next when some manoeuvre is not working. All these thoughts and images run through my thoughts at any time of the day. I have woken at night with pictures of arteries yet to be fixed but awaiting me that morning. This, this is not enjoyable. It is, and has been, a burden. For me, personally, it has been the price I have had to pay for whatever I have achieved. I have not seen any other way to be. I am not an obsessive-compulsive individual. Not even close. Yet in this world of coronary interventions, the room for error is so very, very tiny. The smallest details can matter. The cases that are straightforward never stay with me. There have simply been too many. But the difficult ones are not uncommon. And the flashbacks remain. As the field has progressed with all the advances I have already noted, the anatomy tackled with these techniques has also been more and more complex – and more and more risky. With these, I close my eyes and see the playing field and rehearse. I do not know how else to do it. Do others feel as I do? I don't know.

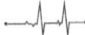

Who could have ever seen all of this happening to me? A guy from the Bronx wanting to be a gym teacher, ending up in Tasmania as an interventional cardiologist, directing a teaching program. There were many, many roadblocks so long ago. Many early failures. Quitting employment halfway through life with no clear idea what was to follow. I really did get lucky. In the cath lab, you also get lucky, but much of that luck is what your skill has brought to you. Moving to Tasmania – that was pure luck. A small advertisement, a few lines in a journal I had no business even looking at. The move was my resurrection and my redemption. Here, at the bottom of the planet, I would find professional success and personal fulfillment. I became one of the fortunate ones. For many years it was not so.

With this book I set out to write stories that would enlighten the public; to have the reader become an 'educated consumer'. I wanted very much to teach something about cardiology and coronary interventions. And to perhaps have the reader gain an understanding at some level about what this life has been like. It is, after all, not the easiest way to make a living. This was not ever meant to be a biography. Yet in the telling of these stories, I have come to realize I could not separate 'me' from the story itself. To do so would have made all this more akin to a textbook. This is not a textbook. It is, I suppose, a memoir of sorts. The arc of my life and how this field, this work, this profession has affected me. It was not my intention when I set out to write.

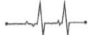

Finally, I sit and write with my thoughts focused on my two sons. It is now decades ago that my fateful decision to come, alone, to the other end of the planet came about. My fork in the road. My sons have nothing to do with this profession. They know very little of these stories that I now so publicly share. I have physically missed much of their adult lives. My 'resurrection' happened without them being here. Their absence has been and has remained … hard. I am so grateful for the advances in telecommunications that allow me now to see them and speak with them regularly. That was not always the case. Not when I first came here. Yet they are on my mind each and every day. Many years ago, I told myself that if I could not be with them physically, I would at least strive to become an example for them of what a man can do if he can overcome his fears and his setbacks. For that really is the tale of my life. This was what I thought I could leave them. What a man can do if he can get past his losses, his failures; to move outside his comfort zone. That is what my fork in the road has been all about. I don't know, will never know I suppose, whether I have accomplished that. I do know that I tried.

So many years ago, it remains clear in my mind. That medical resident who knew what to do when the chips were down. Entered the room, took charge, saved a life. It was then that I knew what I wanted to be. The one to call in difficult moments. The one who wanted 'the ball'. Did I ever become that guy? I guess I will leave that for others to decide. But I do think that in the trying, I became a better man.

ACKNOWLEDGEMENTS

I am not a writer by trade. So there are many to thank, some for their help in putting together the thoughts that ramble through my mind, and some for making my career a semblance of success. I wish to thank Bríd Morahan for helping me in my initial attempts to write a story, guiding me away from a tendency towards a 'textbook' mentality, towards one in which I would allow myself to bring my personal feelings into the narrative. And so many thanks to my publisher and editor, Sue Young, who would guide this tale to fruition with the skill to make my ramblings into a readable account of my life and life's work. My thoughts extend back in time to those early mentors during my time at the University of Pittsburgh, including Drs James Shaver, Barry Uretsky, PS Reddy, Ed Curtis, William Follansbee, Rose Salerno, and Douglas Schulman. Those rare mentors never forgotten.

I cannot forget my forever friend, Dr Bruce Feldman, who was the first singular moment in a series of those 'one things' that would ultimately help me become what it is I have become. And then the second 'one thing' that happened to change the course of my life, my sister Ellen.

I must also thank Dr Rob Fasset, who would take a chance and hire me from across the ocean and allow me the latitude to grow the cardiology program in Launceston, Tasmania. And how could I ever have done without the key players in the department. My first 'trainee', a misnomer if there ever was one, Dr George

Koshy. He made my re-entry back into cardiac care a much easier one. Thank you to Susan Kerkham, my private secretary, banker, provider of lunches and all-rounder, for keeping my private office afloat. Thanks to Jenni Ingles, my secretary in hospital, whose dedication and loyalty were never taken for granted. This would not have happened without her. Thanks to all those advanced trainees and fellows who passed through the department and allowed me to touch the future. And to those in the Cath Lab in those early days, with a special thanks to Sharon Stuart, Shelly Foale, Kirsten Godier, Alex Lendvay, Anita Knight, Nick Merrony, Dario Lokai, Jo Wright and all those others who came when I called. A very special thanks to Mr Robert Miller, my radiographer, friend, and last man standing.

While I remain indebted to those above, who were instrumental in my professional career, I would be delinquent in failing to acknowledge those in my personal life. Thank you to my friends Penny and Richard Price, Joe Tempone and Jenni Wiltshire, Rod Ascui and Kim Seagram, Dr Terry Hannan and Mary Suchodolsky. You reminded me what community is all about when I had lost those feelings many years earlier. To my extended Gordon family, Shari, Verity, Will, and James, who welcomed me into their lives when my own sons were so far away. You have sustained me. Especially the chocolate chip cookies. And the love. To my dear friend Ranju, who has been there since my first days of arrival in Tasmania and to whom I owe a lifelong supply of olive bread. And finally, none of this happens, none of it – the work, the writing, the 'becoming' – without Elizabeth.

GLOSSARY

Angina Symptoms caused by coronary artery blood supply limitations; usually from obstructing plaque accumulation in the artery. Symptoms range from chest tightness or pressure to breathing difficulties.

Angiogram Generic term for pictures of blood vessels obtained following the injection of contrast dye into the circulation.

Angioplasty The term used to describe opening up obstructed blood vessels. Originally performed with balloons, other devices have evolved over time, notably stents.

Balloons In interventions, these are used to open obstructed arteries. They are passed along the guidewire until positioned, then inflated; and removed following deflation, with nothing left in the artery. Of note, inflations are done with a device to calibrate exact pressure ranging from one to twenty-five times atmospheric pressure, with ultrahigh pressure balloons reaching thirty-five times atmospheric pressure.

Blood Pressure (BP) Pressure in the arterial system driving forward flow of blood. 'Top' number is systolic pressure, the maximum pressure obtained following cardiac contraction. 'Bottom' number is diastolic pressure, the minimum pressure occurring during cardiac relaxation.

Burr The 'drill bit' used in rotational atherectomy.

Catheters Long hollow tubes passed through the circulation to their destination, used for the delivery of contrast dye for imaging, and in the case of interventions, used to deliver the equipment, for example stents.

Cath lab Short for (cardiac) catheterization lab. The name of the theatre space where catheters are manipulated into the heart and coronary procedures are performed.

Cardiogenic shock The term used to describe a clinical scenario when the patient has very low blood pressure (i.e. less than 90 mm Hg systolic) and poor cardiac function resulting in poor blood supply to vital organs. Life threatening if not reversed.

Coils In vascular systems, these are delivered to clot off the blood vessel. Named due to the shape of these devices once delivered

Collateral flow Flow to an arterial territory that is totally blocked off, via small channels formed from a second artery. Normally indicative of a chronic problem. The flow delivered is normally not as adequate as the original blood supply, but enough to keep muscle tissue alive.

Dissection A tear in the inner wall of an artery creating a flap-like structure.

Echocardiogram Cardiac ultrasound.

Electrocardiogram (ECG) A tracing of the electrical activity of the heart, usually done by placing a series of wires or 'leads' onto the chest wall and limbs of the body. Instrumental in making the diagnosis of a variety of cardiac conditions which include heart attacks

Guidewires Small wires used to pass through blood vessels. Coronary guidewires are those used to move through coronary vessels and serve as a 'rail' along which balloons and stents can be shuttled in and out.

Intra-aortic balloon pump A large inflatable balloon positioned in the descending aorta, timed to inflate and deflate as the heart relaxes and contracts. Serves to improve coronary and cerebral blood supply in cardiogenic shock. May improve peripheral organ blood flow.

Ischemia Inadequate arterial blood flow to an organ thus depriving it of oxygen and nutrients. In heart disease, classic symptoms include chest pain and breathlessness.

Left anterior descending artery (LAD) One of the three major coronary arteries of the heart, covering much of the anterior heart wall.

Left circumflex artery (LCx) One of the three major coronary arteries of the heart covering the lateral and at times, posterior heart wall.

Left main artery (LM) This is a short artery that 'bifurcates' into the LAD and LCx arteries. The most important bit of vessel architecture in the coronary circulation.

Lucas device A battery powered, pneumatic piston-like pump used to deliver chest compressions during resuscitation. Once turned on, human compression is no longer required.

Lumen The inside of a blood vessel where blood is flowing.

Glossary

Macrovasculature Pertains to arterial blood vessels that can be seen with the naked eye.

Microvasculature Refers to arterial blood vessels that cannot be seen with the naked eye: usually less than 0.3–0.5 mm. Makes up the majority of the arterial circulation throughout all organs.

Open heart surgery also known as bypass surgery, done to improve blood supply to blocked coronary arteries. Requires surgically opening the chest, using other blood vessels in the body to create 'bypasses' around the blockages.

Ostium The origin of the artery.

Percutaneous coronary intervention (PCI) A technique of repairing diseased coronary arteries via a small puncture or incision of the skin (cutaneous). Usually reserved for coronary stenting but may apply to any number of other techniques used to repair coronary vessels. Has essentially replaced the term coronary angioplasty in modern literature.

Pericardiocentesis Technique using aspiration needle directed through the skin into the pericardium for the purpose of fluid removal.

Pericarditis Inflammation of the pericardium. Most commonly viral, although can be secondary to other problems.

Pericardium Sac-like structure surrounding the heart itself.

Right coronary artery (RCA) One of the three major coronary arteries covering the inferior and at times, posterior heart wall.

Rotational atherectomy Use of a high-speed rotating drill or burr to open calcified arteries. Rotating speeds vary and go as high as 200,000 rpm.

Stents Used to open obstructions, scaffolding the vessels open. Made of various metallic alloys. Delivered crimped onto a balloon. Once expanded, the stent is left in the artery while the delivery balloon is removed. Once expanded, stents are not retrievable.

Tamponade The physiology created when fluid accumulates in the pericardium, causing 'squeezing' of the heart muscle itself, thus limiting its ability to fill adequately with returning blood flow. While tamponade exists on a continuum, when causing low blood pressure, it is life threatening.

Valvular insufficiency /regurgitation Leaking heart valves. Range from trivial to severe.

www.ingramcontent.com/pod-product-compliance
Lightning Source LLC
Chambersburg PA
CBHW021059080526
44587CB00010B/308